Current Practices in Ophthalmology

Series Editor

Parul Ichhpujani
Department of Ophthalmology
Government Medical College and Hospital
Chandigarh, India

This series of highly organized and uniform handbooks aims to cover the latest clinically relevant developments in ophthalmology. In the wake of rapidly evolving innovations in the field of basic research, pharmacology, surgical techniques and imaging devices for the management of ophthalmic disorders, it is extremely important to invest in books that help you stay updated. These handbooks are designed to bridge the gap between journals and standard texts providing reviews on advances that are now part of mainstream clinical practice. Meant for residents, fellows-in-training, generalist ophthalmologists and specialists alike, each volume under this series covers current perspectives on relevant topics and meets the CME requirements as a go-to reference guide. Supervised and reviewed by a subject expert(s), chapters in each volume provide leading-edge information most relevant and useful for clinical ophthalmologists. This series is also useful for residents and fellows training in various subspecialties of ophthalmology, who can read these books while at work or during emergency duties. Additionally, these handbooks can aid in preparing for clinical case discussions at various forums and examinations.

More information about this series at http://www.springer.com/series/15743

Parul Ichhpujani • Sahil Thakur

Smart Resources in Ophthalmology

Applications and Social Networking

Springer

Parul Ichhpujani
Department of Ophthalmology
Government Medical College and Hospital
Chandigarh
India

Sahil Thakur
Department of Ophthalmology
Government Medical College and Hospital
Chandigarh
India

ISSN 2523-3807 ISSN 2523-3815 (electronic)
Current Practices in Ophthalmology
ISBN 978-981-13-0139-1 ISBN 978-981-13-0140-7 (eBook)
https://doi.org/10.1007/978-981-13-0140-7

Library of Congress Control Number: 2018942949

Printed on acid-free paper

This Springer imprint is published by the registered company Springer Nature Singapore Pte Ltd. part of Springer Nature
The registered company address is: 152 Beach Road, #21-01/04 Gateway East, Singapore 189721, Singapore

Preface

"A poem begins with a lump in the throat… It is a reaching-out toward expression; an effort to find fulfilment. A complete poem is one where an emotion has found its thought and the thought has found words."

Robert Frost's lines can be easily adopted as our own. This book is an expression of emotions that we have felt everyday while seeing the patients in the hospital. Can we do something innovative that makes their and our life easier? Mobile technology was the quickest avenue that gave us answers. As mobile data search applications on the Android/iOS platforms are fast replacing all the libraries of the world, it is imperative that we capitalize on this 'app' boom. We tried to find resources that could guide us in this massive conundrum of countless applications but sadly couldn't find one that could aid us in this journey. We sincerely hope none of you have to feel that way when you look at the treasure trove of applications currently available on your mobile devices. The book can additionally help you streamline and optimize your current practice. We have also included user-friendly applications like drug/revisit reminders that you can suggest to your patients and in turn make sure that they come back to you for future referrals. We have also included useful social media and website links which we feel can add to this connected experience. After all who doesn't want a doctor who is just a few clicks away? We specifically added the QR codes for each application to make this experience a truly interactive one. It is most emphatically not a substitute for a detailed clinical examination. This book is a humble attempt to guide you, inspire you and above all to help you download the application that you always wanted but never knew existed.

Best wishes and Happy Downloading!!

Chandigarh, India

Parul Ichhpujani
Sahil Thakur

Contents

About the Authors

Parul Ichhpujani is currently an Associate Professor at the Department of Ophthalmology, Government Medical College and Hospital, Chandigarh, India, where she is responsible for the glaucoma and neuro-ophthalmology services. She completed her glaucoma training at the Advanced Eye Centre, Postgraduate Institute of Medical Education and Research, Chandigarh, India, followed by a clinical research fellowship under Dr George L. Spaeth at Wills Eye Institute, Philadelphia, USA. She is an avid researcher and academic. She has co-authored a book, *Pearls in Glaucoma Therapy*; edited three books, *Expert Techniques in Ophthalmology*, *Manual of Glaucoma* and *Glaucoma: Basic and Clinical Perspectives*; and contributed several research articles and book chapters in national as well as international books. Dr. Ichhpujani has lectured at regional, national and international surgical meetings and serves as a reviewer for various ophthalmology journals. She was named in the power list of "*Best 40 under 40*" ophthalmologists in 2014.

Sahil Thakur is a budding ophthalmologist who, apart from pursuing clinical aspects of ophthalmology, has a keen interest in affordable medical technology and clinical photography. His presentations at various scientific fora were evidence-based studies done using smartphone apps or online tools for ophthalmic investigations. He is currently involved in research and development of digital software for faster and more efficient diagnosis of common ophthalmic disorders. He is following his mentor Dr Parul Ichhpujani's footsteps into the field of medical books.

What Is a "Smart" Device? 1

A smart device is an electronic device, connected to other devices or networks via different wireless protocols such as Bluetooth, near-field communication (NFC), Wi-Fi, 3G, 4G, etc. that have the ability to operate interactively and autonomously. Currently available smart devices include smartphones, tablets and phablets, smart bands, smart watches and smart key chains. Most commonly used among the smart devices are the smartphones.

On April 3, 1973, Martin Cooper, a Motorola employee, made the first mobile handheld cellular telephone call in New York City. Since then cellular phones have evolved into small wireless computers with Bluetooth and Internet connectivity, thus appropriately labelled as *smartphones*. The smartphones have virtually invaded our personal and professional space.

There are a few key components necessary for a mobile phone handset to be a *smartphone*:

- It should be designed for personal use rather than designed for business or commercial use.
- It should have the ability to connect to the Internet in a constant, unrestricted way.
- It should have the ability to install a range of applications (apps) from an external source, such as an 'app store'.
- It should have a high-resolution screen and a high-definition camera to facilitate high-quality video conferencing and image acquisition capability [1].

Smartphones have taken the world by storm primarily due to the ease of wireless mobile computing that they offer. Every day the technology behind smart devices gets even smarter making them an indispensable part of our lives. The number of smartphone users is predicted to grow from 3.2 billion in 2015 to around 6.3 billion in 2021, with smartphone penetration rates increasing exponentially as well [2].

P. Ichhpujani, S. Thakur, *Smart Resources in Ophthalmology*, Current Practices in Ophthalmology, https://doi.org/10.1007/978-981-13-0140-7_1

Tablets and Phablets

A **tablet computer** or **"tablet"** is a mobile personal computer. The hardware and software that make the tablet work are housed in a single thin flat package. Ever since Issac Assimov described a fictional prototype in his novel Foundation, mobile computing has today come a long way. Based on operating systems like iOS, Android, Ubuntu Touch and Windows, tablets bring the easy accessibility of smartphones and powerful processing/screen size of desktop computers together in a functional and versatile package. With the ability to add accessories like keyboard, stylus and VR devices to the tablet platform, we today have a device that has potentially limitless flexibility. This is why tablets are so popular devices for medical use [3–5]. Recently, a new generation of devices have made the mobile computing market even more interesting. Smartphones with screen sizes between 5.5 in. (140 mm) and 7 in. (180 mm) and an aspect ratio of 16:9 have blurred the borders between tablets and smartphones. These 'phablet' devices offer app developers more screen size to work with while maintaining the easy accessibility of the smartphone form factor.

Smart Device Use by Doctors: Pros and Cons

The usage of smart devices by doctors has also been increasing day by day. A survey in Ireland showed that 94.4% of junior doctors own a smartphone and on at least a daily basis used it for the purposes of work, 83.3% made or received phone calls, 87.2% sent or received texts, 52.9% used their smartphone to take work-related pictures, and 41.2% sent or received emails on their smartphone [6]. Similarly high percentage of smartphone usage has been reported elsewhere [7, 8].

Ophthalmological applications are today widely available across operating systems and can turn smartphones into sophisticated medical devices. They are useful tools for the practice of evidence-based medicine, professional and patient education, mobile clinical communication, disease self-management, remote patient monitoring or as powerful administrative tools [9]. There are also several applications that are available for different ophthalmological examinations that can assess visual acuity, colour vision, astigmatism, pupil size, Amsler grid test and more [10]. Smartphones in conjunction with a +20D lens or external attachments can be used for taking images of anterior and posterior eye segment that are comparable to those taken with expensive fundus/anterior segment cameras [11, 12].

Many physicians have raised concerns about the inappropriate use of the cell phones/smartphones in letters to the editors of various academic journals and online surveys. In a 2015 survey, vast majority of the doctors (95.2%) endorsed use of smartphone. Nearly all (97.1%) carried a cell phone with them at work. While at work, only 6.3% kept their phones in silent mode, while 72.1% and 21.6% left their phones on vibrate and ring mode, respectively. Approximately half of them (56.7%) password protected their cell phone. Participants were also asked to rate how much they relied on their phones on a scale from 1 (not at all) to 5 (can't leave home without it). Most individuals (91.9%) rated their reliance a 4 (31.3%) or 5 (60.6%). The study further showed how doctors don't consider their usage unprofessional but find patient usage of phone during an interaction highly irritable [13].

With the increased utility of social networking applications like WhatsApp for professional interaction, ethical issues of ownership of data, security of confidential information and need of patient consent for transmission over Internet via these applications have also cropped up [14]. What is more alarming to note is the possibility of transmission of pathogens due to the excessive use of smartphones. In a recent study, 96.2% mobile phones were contaminated with bacteria [15]. Such microbiological data is adding up every day, and in the future it is possible that hospital administrations across the world will come forward with tougher protocols to deal with the usage of smartphones in critical areas like the intensive care units and admission wards.

We are sure of the fact that smartphones and their usage in medicine are here to stay, more so in branches like ophthalmology that are so dependent on image acquisition and its interpretation. With their expanding use into screening the population for diabetes, glaucoma and other ocular pathologies, the utility of smartphones outweighs their shortcomings [12, 16, 17]. This book is an attempt to make sense out of the several 'apps' that are available to an ophthalmologist on their phone today and how they can easily integrate them into their clinical practice. We have enough evidence how mobile applications can enhance the safety, efficiency, effectiveness and timeliness of patient care [18]. Some authors even mention that phones have become as essential to a doctor as a stethoscope, and this statement only underlines the role that smartphones will have in patient care in the future [19]. Till we have a clearer understanding of mobile etiquette and consensus-based guidelines to use mobile phones at work are framed, all we can do is to keep up with the wireless revolution by clicking, downloading and healing.

References

1. Nasser FB, Trevena L. There's an app for that: a guide for healthcare practitioners and researchers on smartphone technology. Online J Public Health Inform. 2015;7(2):e218.
2. Ericsson Mobility Report 2016 [cited 2017]. https://www.ericsson.com/mobility-report
3. Nesaratnam N, Thomas PBM, Kirollos R, Vingrys AJ, Kong GYX, Martin KR. Tablets at the bedside—iPad-based visual field test used in the diagnosis of Intrasellar Haemangiopericytoma: a case report. BMC Ophthalmol. 2017;17(1):53.
4. Rosen PN, Boer ER, Barbosa Gracitelli CP, Abe RY, Diniz-Filho A, Marvasti A, et al. Visual performance assessment using a mobile platform. Investig Ophthalmol Vis Sci. 2015;56(7):3177.
5. Holmes JM, Manh VM, Lazar EL, Beck RW, Birch EE, Kraker RT, et al. Effect of a Binocular iPad Game vs Part-Time Patching in children aged 5 to 12 years with amblyopia: a randomized clinical trial. JAMA Ophthalmol. 2016;134(12):1391–400.
6. O'Connor P, Byrne D, Butt M, Offiah G, Lydon S, Mc Inerney K, et al. Interns and their smartphones: use for clinical practice. Postgrad Med J. 2014;90(1060):75–9.
7. Payne KFB, Wharrad H, Watts K. Smartphone and medical related App use among medical students and junior doctors in the United Kingdom (UK): a regional survey. BMC Med Inform Decis Mak. 2012;12(1):121.

8. Katz-Sidlow RJ, Ludwig A, Miller S, Sidlow R. Smartphone use during inpatient attending rounds: prevalence, patterns and potential for distraction. J Hosp Med. 2012;7(8):595–9.
9. Zvornicanin E, Zvornicanin J, Hadziefendic B. The use of smart phones in ophthalmology. Acta Inform Med. 2014;22(3):206–9.
10. Chhablani J, Kaja S, Shah VA. Smartphones in ophthalmology. Indian J Ophthalmol. 2012;60(2):127–31.
11. Bastawrous A. Smartphone fundoscopy. Ophthalmology. 2012;119(2):432–3.e2.
12. Bastawrous A, Giardini ME, Bolster NM, Peto T, Shah N, Livingstone IA, et al. Clinical validation of a smartphone-based adapter for optic disc imaging in Kenya. JAMA Ophthalmol. 2016;134(2):151–8.
13. Johnson AC, El Hajj SC, Perret JN, Caffery TS, Jones GN, Musso MW. Smartphones in medicine: emerging practices in an academic medical center. J Med Syst. 2015;39(1):164.
14. Natarajan S, Nair AG. Outsmarted by the smartphone! Indian J Ophthalmol. 2015;63(10):757–8.
15. Zakai S, Mashat A, Abumohssin A, Samarkandi A, Almaghrabi B, Barradah H, et al. Bacterial contamination of cell phones of medical students at King Abdulaziz University, Jeddah, Saudi Arabia. J Microsc Ultrastruct. 2016;4(3):143–6.
16. Furdova A, Furdova A, Krcmery V. Our experience with smartphone and spherical lens for the eye fundus examination during humanitarian project in Africa. Int J Ophthalmol. 2017;10(1):157–60.
17. Bolster NM, Giardini ME, Bastawrous A. The diabetic retinopathy screening workflow: potential for smartphone imaging. J Diabetes Sci Technol. 2015;10(2):318–24.
18. Webb K, Bullock A, Dimond R, Stacey M. Can a mobile app improve the quality of patient care provided by trainee doctors? Analysis of trainees' case reports. BMJ Open. 2016;6(9):e013075.
19. Dimond R, Bullock A, Lovatt J, Stacey M. Mobile learning devices in the workplace: 'as much a part of the junior doctors' kit as a stethoscope'? BMC Med Educ. 2016;16(1):207.

Apps and Social Networking Pages for Basic Workup

2

Many ophthalmologists need to perform consultation and examination in emergency rooms where ophthalmic test equipments are not readily available. With the advent of smart devices, several basic vision tests can now be carried at the patient's bedside in emergency room or outside the clinic. Additionally, patients with some ocular diseases, such as age-related macular degeneration, can also use their smartphones to perform regular checks between office visits for timely detection of any change.

Apps for oculo-visual system are available both on iOS platform and Google Android store. iOS does not traditionally support older apps once a newer version of the operating system becomes available. This contrasts with Google Android, where older apps may remain available to users in the marketplace unless they are manually removed by the app developer.

Smartphone Applications

This chapter will broadly address some basic vision testing applications under the following heads:

A. Apps for Visual acuity assessment and Refraction
B. Apps for Color Vision testing
C. Apps for Amsler grid testing
D. Apps for Pupil assessment
E. Apps for Contrast sensitivity
F. Apps for Physician training

A. **Apps for Visual Acuity Assessment**
   Accurate visual acuity assessment is quintessential to the workup of any patient with visual complaints, especially those presenting in the emergency settings.

P. Ichhpujani, S. Thakur, *Smart Resources in Ophthalmology*, Current Practices in Ophthalmology, https://doi.org/10.1007/978-981-13-0140-7_2

Precise visual acuity assessment using Snellen test depends on how much effort and confidence the patient puts in to read the alphabets and whether the patient is wearing a recently obtained refractive correction (glasses or contact lenses). The emergency staff is most of the times not formally trained in ophthalmic examination and hence may not understand the nuances of administering the Snellen test.

Studies have shown that vision measured by non-ophthalmic emergency department staff with a mobile app is more accurate than with a Snellen chart [1]. Therefore, such apps may serve as a valuable tool for non-ophthalmic emergency department staff.

1. ***Eye Chart Pro***
   - ***Platforms***: iPad (Free)
   - ***App Creator***: Dok LLC (Manu Lakkur)
   - ***Version***: 2.0.4
   - ***App Size***: 24 MB
   - ***App Icon***:

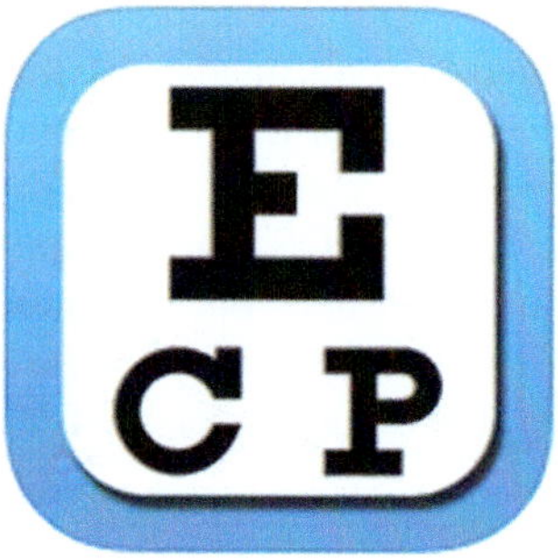

   - ***App Screenshots***:

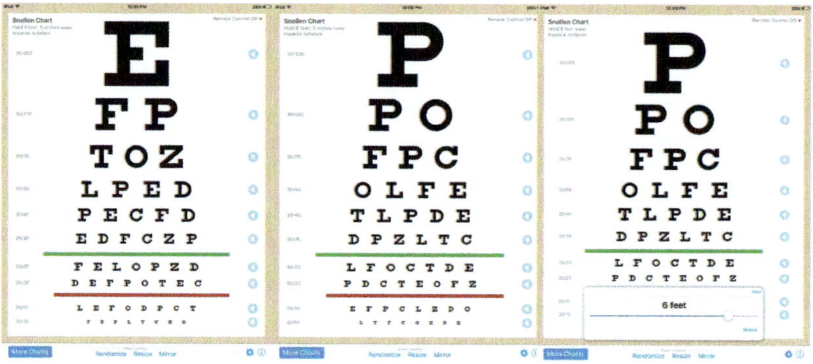

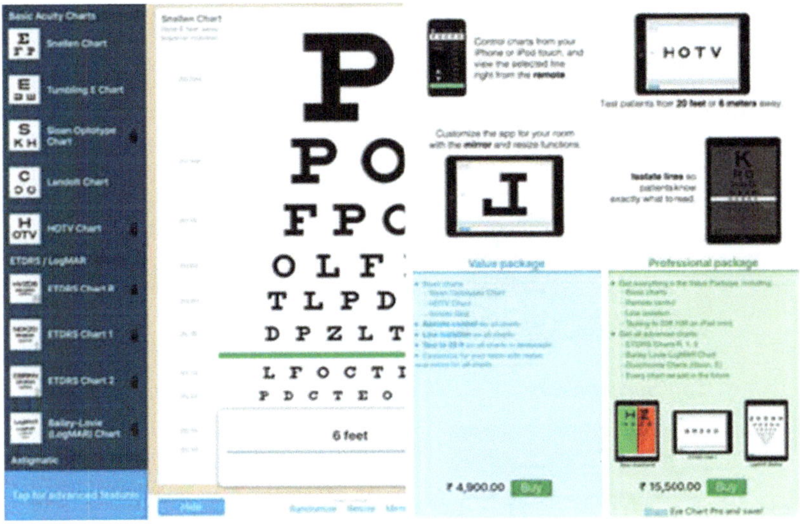

- ***Features***:
  Eye Chart Pro is a randomizable visual acuity tool. User can easily toggle between Snellen and Tumbling E chart. It is useful for triaging and house visits and especially for patients who memorize the office chart. Zhang and coworkers reported that the Eye Chart Pro iOS app was a reliable method for testing distance visual acuity in outpatient, only when the Snellen visual acuity was better than 20/200 [2].
- ***QR Scanning Code for the App***

2. ***Eye Chart Professional***
   - ***Platforms***: iPad
   - ***App Creator***: Dok LLC (Manu Lakkur)
   - ***Version***: 2.0.1
   - ***App Size***: 22.1 MB

- ***App Icon***:

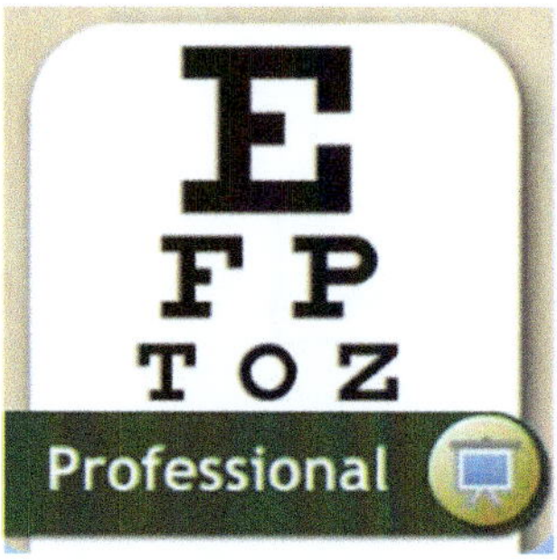

- ***App Screenshots***:

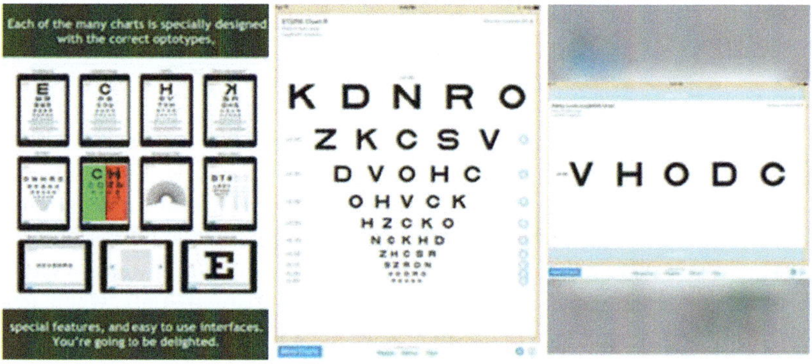

- ***Features***:
  This app is appropriate for house visits by the doctor, hospital bedside testing or mounted to a wall as an upgrade to eye chart projector.

  QR Scanning Codes for the App

3. ***Eye Chart Pro Remote Control***
   - ***Platforms***: iPhone
   - ***App Creator***: Dok LLC (Manu Lakkur)
   - ***Version***: 2.0

- ***App Size***: 2.3 MB
- ***App Icon***:

- ***App Screenshots***:

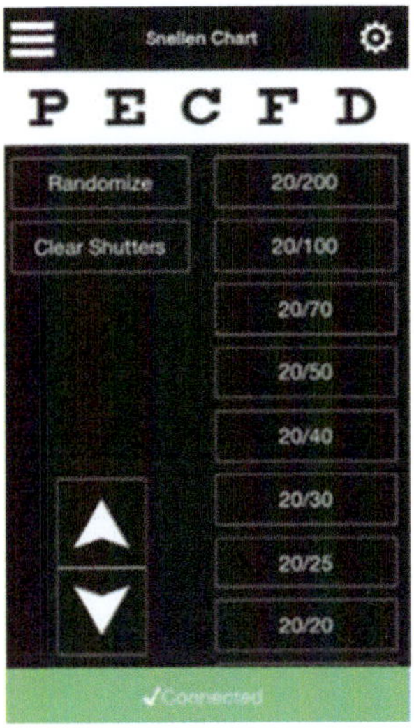

- ***Features***:
  This app works in tandem with the Eye Chart Pro, Eye Chart Premium and Eye Chart Professional apps on the iPad, as the remote control.

  QR Scanning Codes for the App

4. ***eyeTests Easy***
   - ***Platforms***: iPad, iPhone, iPod Touch (Free; English, Japanese)
   - ***App Creator***: George Kong Softwares
   - ***Version***: 8.0
   - ***App Size***: 13.7 MB
   - ***App Icon***:

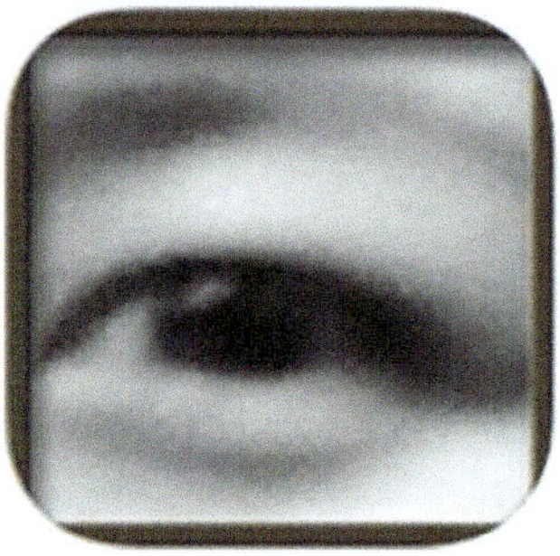

   - ***App Screenshots***:

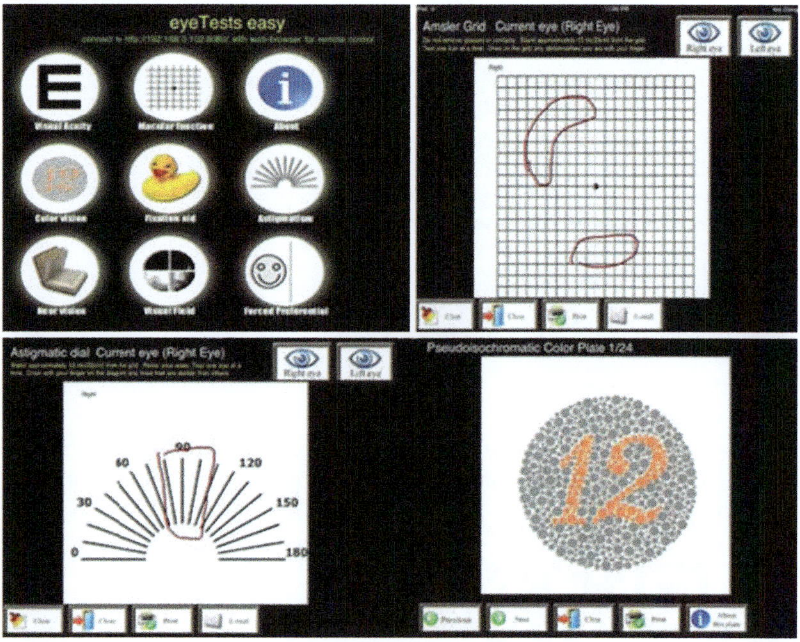

   - ***Features***:
     This app tests several parameters including distance and near visual acuity, colour vision, macular function and peripheral vision. Hence, it is useful not only for ophthalmologists but also general practitioners, optometrists, opticians and even patients. The scrolling of visual acuity chart can be done using any mobile phone device or laptop using Wi-Fi. The viewing distance can be adjusted for distance and near (6 m, 3 m, 1.2 m and 40 cm).

In preverbal children, forced preferential looking test can be done by following the child's gaze, on projecting engaging cartoon images. Clinicians can also maintain child's fixation using these cartoon images. It also allows free-hand drawing onto colour plates to outline the projected number or shape.

The app also allows monitoring of macular function using a standard Amsler grid. Patients can chart any abnormalities in their macular vision on the Amsler grid using a finger, and the Amsler grid images can then be emailed to their clinician.

Peripheral vision is tested using suprathreshold method.

The app can test near acuity from N18 to N5.

Note: When any device or tool is used for measuring near visual acuity, it must be calibrated for use at 36 cm and represent similar number of characters and distance between the characters themselves within each line equated to the conventional near cards. The difference in the contrast ratios of the high-definition smartphone screens (with variable screen technology, resolution, size and pixel density) and the near vision cards may result in some discrepancies of the measured near acuity [3].

QR Scanning Code for the App

5. ***Smart Optometry***
   - ***Platforms***: iPhone, iPad, Android
   - ***App Creator***: Smart Optometry d.o.o
   - ***Version***: 3.5
   - ***App Size***: 114 MB (iOS); 30.9MB (Android)
   - ***App Icon***:

- ***App Screenshots***:

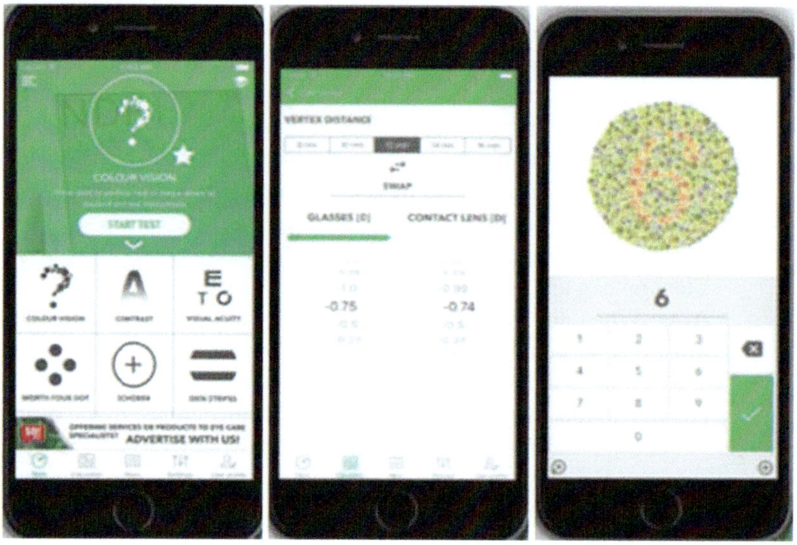

- ***Features***:
  Smart Optometry includes 16 ophthalmic tests including colour vision, contrast sensitivity, visual acuity, worth four dot, Schober, OKN stripes, fluorescein light, red desaturation, Hirschberg, accommodation, duochrome test, aniseikonia, Amsler grid, MEM retinoscopy, maze for amblyopia test and visual acuity +. The app also has a vertex conversion calculator and a visual acuity conversion calculator. This app is available in 11 languages.

  QR Scanning Code for the App

  iOS Android

6. ***Eye Test-Eye Exam***
   - ***Platforms***: Android
   - ***App Creator***: healthcare4mobile
   - ***Version***: 1.1.0
   - ***App Size***: 6.5MB

- ***App Icon***:

- ***App Screenshots***:

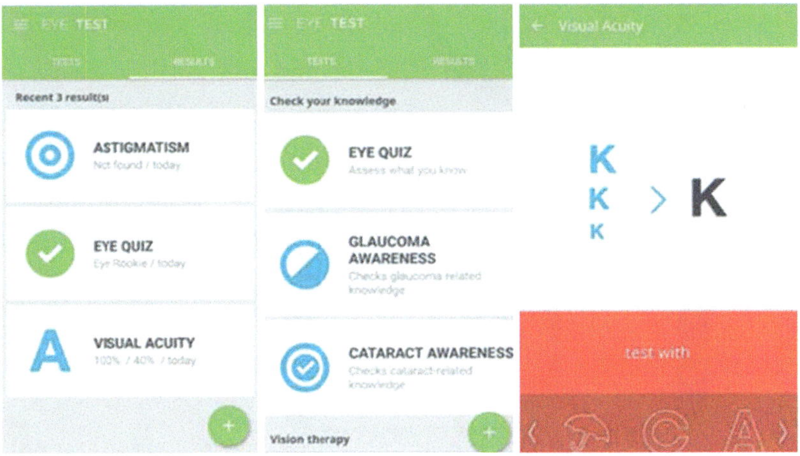

- ***Features***:
  The app has 12 ophthalmic tests that help assess visual acuity (based on standard charts such as Snellen chart, LogMAR chart, Golovin-Sivtsev table, Landolt C/Japanese Vision Test, Tumbling E chart) and colour perception disturbances and helps screen for accommodation spasm, dry eye, cataracts and macular degeneration. Additionally, it also has eight eye health quizzes to see if the user knows about the common vision-related or ocular problems.

  QR Scanning Code for the App

7. ***Peek Acuity***
   - ***Platforms***: Android (English, French and Spanish)
   - ***App Creator***: Peek Vision
   - ***Version***: 3.5.0
   - ***App Size***: 24 MB
   - ***App Icon***:

   - ***App Screenshots***:

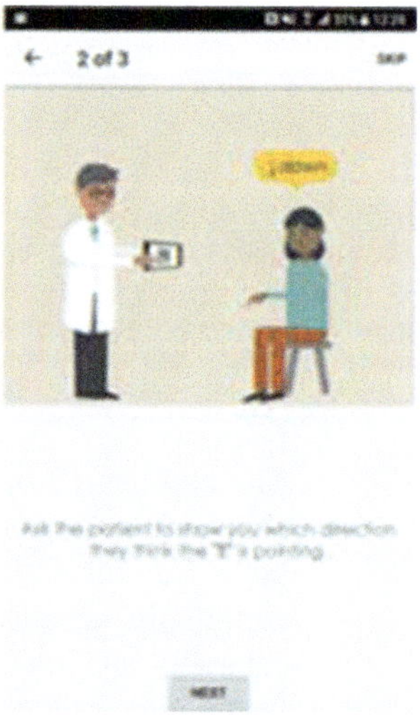

   - ***Features***:
     This ETDRS visual acuity-based app generates visual acuity scores in standard units of Snellen [both metric (6/6) and imperial (20/20) values] and LogMAR (0.0). It also includes equivalents of 'count fingers', 'hand movement' and 'light perception' and a simulated representation that helps explain those scores to patients.
     The app uses only the letter 'E' in four orientations. The examinee points in the direction of the arms of the E, and the examiner records the response

by swiping across the screen in the same direction. The app is smart as it senses ambient light and automatically adjusts screen brightness. If the surroundings are too bright for accurate measurements, the examiner is alerted.

Bastawrous et al. validated the Peek Acuity app against Snellen charts and a clinic measurement using the ETDRS chart as part of an epidemiologic eye survey in central Kenya [4]. The investigators found the use of their app took almost similar time as Snellen vision testing and concluded that the app was repeatable and consistent.

Peek Acuity Pro: This is a CE-registered class 1 medical device available in countries where it is registered for use (UK and Ireland).

QR Scanning Code for the App

8. ***Optics Clinical Calculator***
   - ***Platforms***: iPhone, iPad, iPod Touch (English, Italian, Portuguese)
   - ***App Creator***: Evan Schoenberg
   - ***Version***: 3.5.0
   - ***App Size***: 24 MB
   - ***App Icon***:

- ***App Screenshots***:

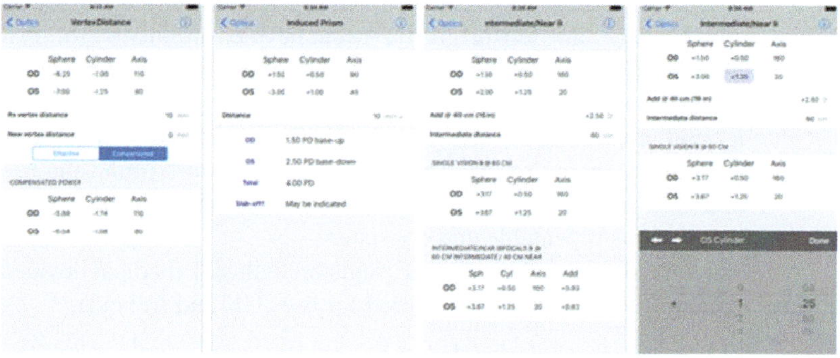

- ***Features***:
  This is a comprehensive calculator application including calculators for several parameters including base curve, diopter conversion to millimetres, diopters from focal distance, convergence, intermediate and near vision prescriptions from standard refraction, lens power in oblique meridians, oblique crossed cylinders, ocular curve, optical centre decentration, slab-off calculator (induced prism) and vertex distance.

  QR Scanning Code for the App

  Note: There are more than 100 vision assessment apps in the Google Play Store and iTunes Store, but only a few have been robustly validated in scientific settings. Therefore, it is prudent to remember that these apps are not a substitute for a clinical examination at the ophthalmologist's clinic but just a broad guide of the functioning of the visual system. One must always remember that individual handsets vary in size and resolution (720p, 1080p and 1440p displays), requiring users to calculate and adapt appropriate distance between the examiner and patient.

B. **Apps for Colour Vision Testing**

Congenital colour vision deficiency affects around 8% of men and 0.4% of women across the world. In addition to the importance of recognizing colours in day-to-day life, for example, looking at traffic signals, maps or graphs, many aspects of health (e.g. change in colour of urine) and healthcare (e.g. colour-coded diagnostic tests, coloured medication pills or coloured medication bottle caps) depend upon colour coding.

Recently, a study has shown dyschromatopsia testing for optic neuritis using a commercially available application on an iPad was comparable to using the pseudo-isochromatic plates of Ishihara [5].

Some of the apps that test for colour vision deficiency have been mentioned in the previous section such as eyeTests Easy, Smart Optometry and Eye Test-Eye Exam which also assess colour vision in addition to other parameters.

Users of smartphone application testing for colour vision deficiency must remember that some apps may have different sensitivity for detection of colour vision deficiency compared to Ishihara booklet, limiting their usefulness for clinical use [6].

1. ***ColorBlindness SimulateCorrect***
   - ***Platforms***: Android
   - ***App Creator***: Seewald Solutions
   - ***Version***: 1.562
   - ***App Size***: 54.6KB
   - ***App Icon***:

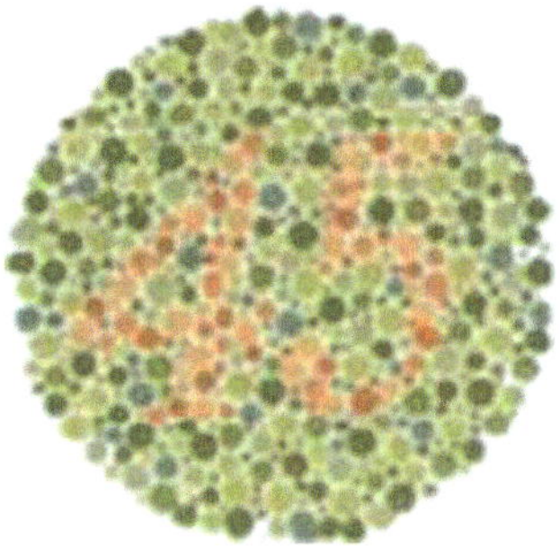

- ***App Screenshot***:

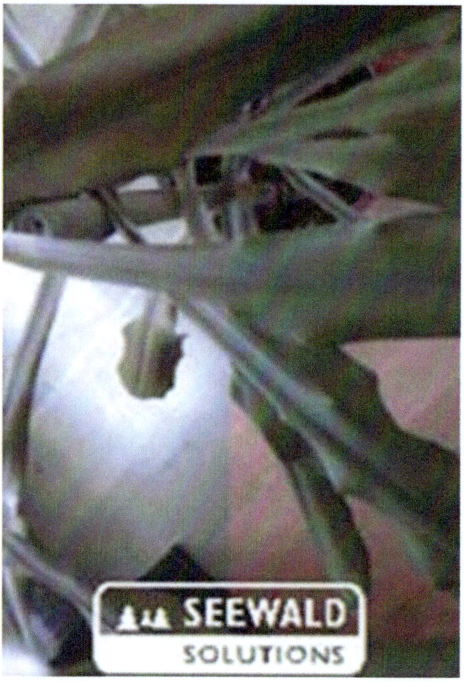

- ***Features***:
  This simple augmented reality application uses the integrated camera of the smartphone to simulate and correct colour blindness in real time. Not only are all common forms of colour blindness supported, but it is also possible to compare with normal vision.

  QR Scanning Code for the App

2. ***Color Blind Pal***
   - ***Platforms***: iPhone, iPad, Android
   - ***App Creator***: Vincent Fiorentini

- ***Version***: 1.0.2
- ***App Size***: 1.6 MB
- ***App Icon***:

- ***App Screenshots***:

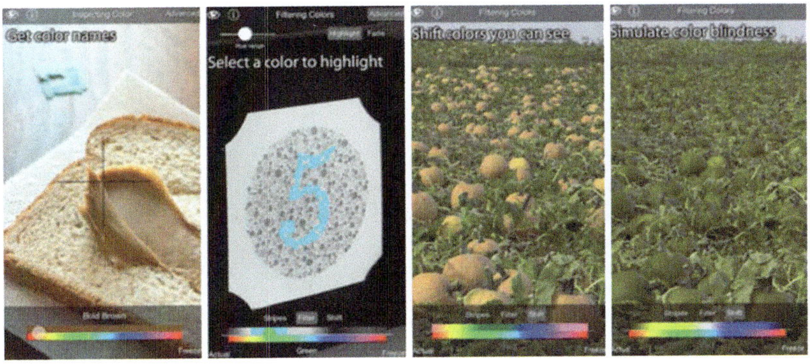

- ***Features***:

  Color Blind Pal helps to find out what is the exact colour of an object and helps to read any colour-coded map, chart or graph. Basically the app has two modes: ‘Inspecting Color’ or ‘Filtering Colors’.

  The ‘Inspecting Color Mode’ helps the user to choose between different types of names for a colour, including common names, colloquial names and scientific names. It also helps to see the colour’s hue, saturation and its exact RGB colour code.

  The ‘Filtering Color Mode’ highlights a selected colour. One can select a colour by pressing it on the screen or by dragging the colour spectrum slider. The app draws a stripe pattern over all reddish colours so one can tell what colour everything is without changing the actual colours. There is an option to freeze the camera and experiment with different filters to get an exact sense of what the image really looks like.

QR Scanning Code for the App

iOS Android

3. ***Color Binoculars, A Microsoft Garage Project***
    - ***Platforms***: iPhone, iPad, iPod Touch
    - ***App Creator***: Microsoft Corporation
    - ***Version***: 1.0.11
    - ***App Size***: 15.4 MB
    - ***App Icon***:
    - ***App Screenshots***:

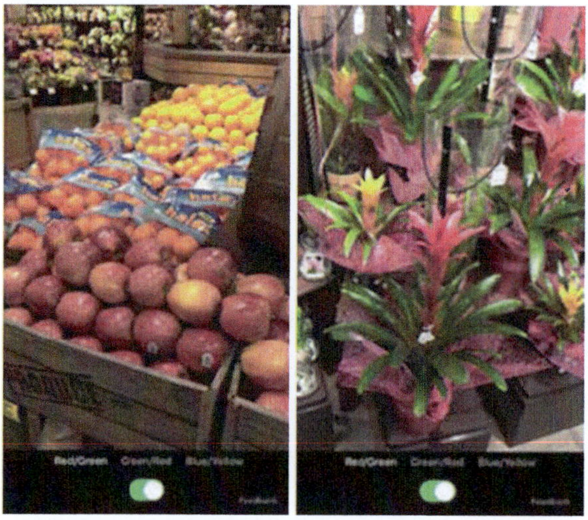

- ***Features***:
  This app has been made by two Microsoft engineers; one of them is colour-blind. Color Binoculars uses the iPhone camera to adjust the colours that one sees to replace difficult colour combinations, like red and green, with a more easily distinguishable combinations, like pink and green. This app supports all three common forms of colour blindness. The app specially comes in handy for day-to-day activities such as choosing matching outfits, picking up flowers, etc.

  QR Scanning Code for the App

4. ***Chromatic Glass***
   - ***Platforms***: iPhone, iPad, iPod Touch (Free; English and Japanese)
   - ***App Creator***: Kazunori Asada
   - ***Version***: 2.16
   - ***App Size***: 13.7 MB
   - ***App Icon***:

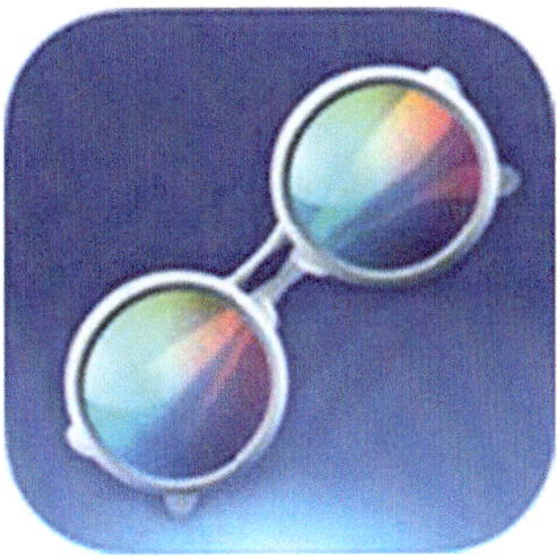

- ***App Screenshots***:

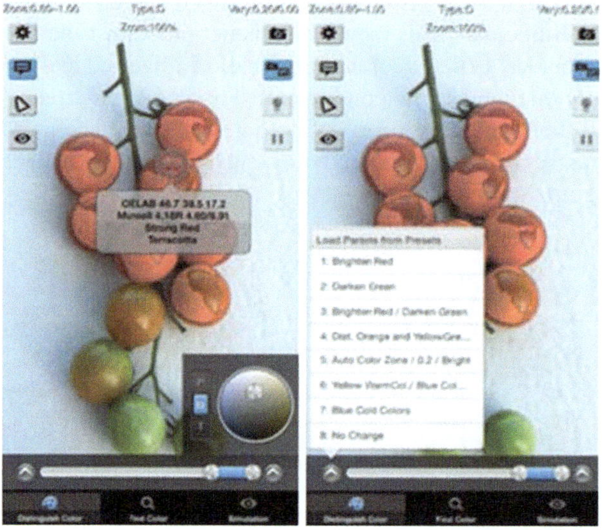

- ***Features***:

  Protans have difficulty in perceiving differences between red, especially deep red. Tritans have difficulty distinguishing between green and blue. This app helps users to recognize and distinguish colours by making a special modified colour image based on scientific theoretical methods in real time and displaying it and the original image alternately.

  QR Scanning Code for the App

C. **Apps for Amsler Grid Testing**

Amsler grid is one of the simplest tools to screen for age-related macular degeneration. There are many apps that have Amsler grid available on the go; some of these have been covered in the first section, such as eyeTests Easy, Smart Optometry and Eye Test-Eye Exam. These apps will also be covered in the section on retinal disorders.

D. **Apps for Pupil Assessment**

Examining the immediate response of the pupil to light stimuli can give an insight in the dysfunctions of autonomic nervous system. Clinically, pupillary light reflex examination utilizes medical penlight to provide the light stimuli at the pupil of the examined person. Not many apps exist to aid in assessment of pupillary light reflex.

1. ***Pupil Scan***
   - ***Platforms***: iPhone, iPad, iPod Touch (Free)
   - ***App Creator***: Brian Wiley
   - ***Version***: 0.6.0
   - ***App Size***: 26.5 MB
   - ***App Icon***:

   - ***App Screenshots***:

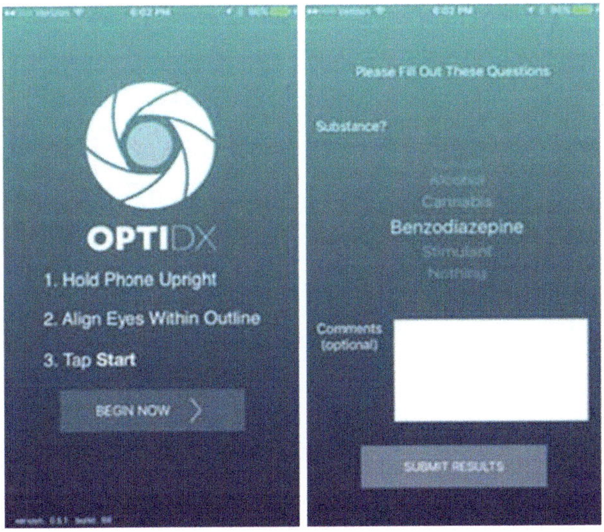

- ***Features***:
  This app records a 3-s-long video, with brief pulses of light directed at the retina, and stores the results. There is also a brief survey at the end to provide some insight on your current state during the recording.

  QR Scanning Code for the App

2. ***Eye MD***
   - ***Platforms***: iPhone, iPad, iPod Touch (Free)
   - ***App Creator***: Code-Red-I LLC
   - ***Version***: 2.0
   - ***App Size***: 21.8 MB
   - ***App Icon***:

   - ***App Screenshot***:

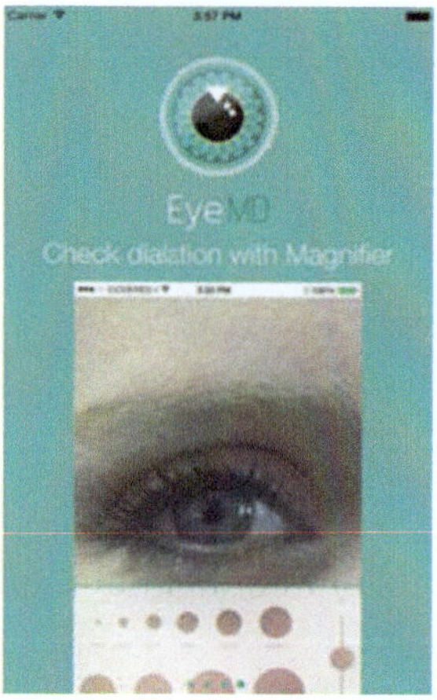

- ***Features***:
  In addition to a magnifier eye exam tool and pupil chart, this app also offers visual acuity assessment, a penlight tool and Ishihara colour test to examine colour blindness.

  QR Scanning Codes for the App

3. ***Pupilometer Free***
   - ***Platforms***: Android (Free)
   - ***App Creator***: Theia
   - ***Version***: 1.2
   - ***App Size***: 247 KB
   - ***App Icon***:

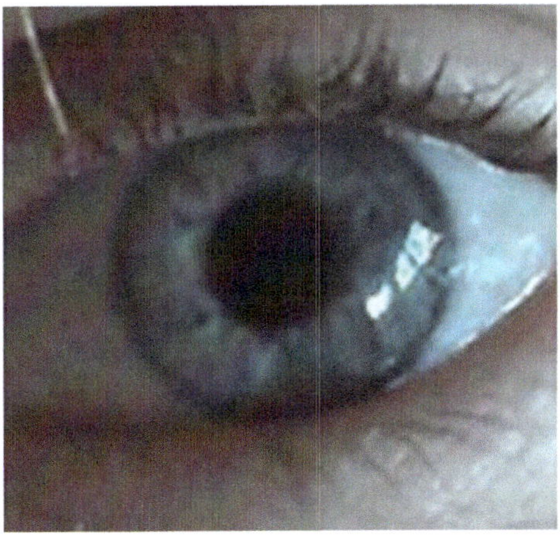

- ***App Screenshots***:

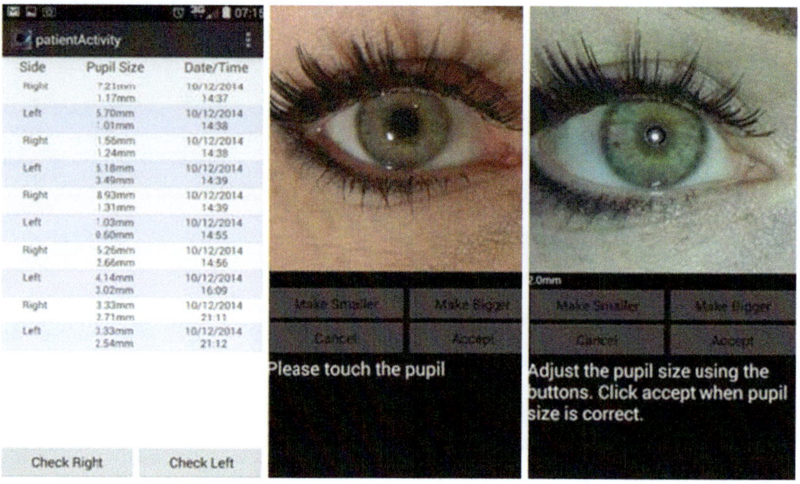

- ***Features***:
  This app is a good tool for nurses, doctors, emergency assistants and medical students to accurately measure a patient's pupil size and reactivity. The app records the pupil size and reactivity along with the date and time and the patients' room number.

  QR Scanning Code for the App

E. **Apps for Contrast Sensitivity**
   Contrast refers to the darkness of the object compared to the lightness of the background. The highest quality print may have 85–95% contrast. Significant loss of contrast sensitivity is common among low-vision patients secondary to pathologies such as advanced diabetic retinopathy, glaucoma and neurological disease.

1. ***Variable Contrast Sensitivity Chart by King Devick***
   - ***Platforms***: iPhone, iPad, iPod Touch
   - ***App Creator***: King Devick Test, LLC

- ***Version***: 2.0
- ***App Size***: 9.4 MB
- ***App Icon***:

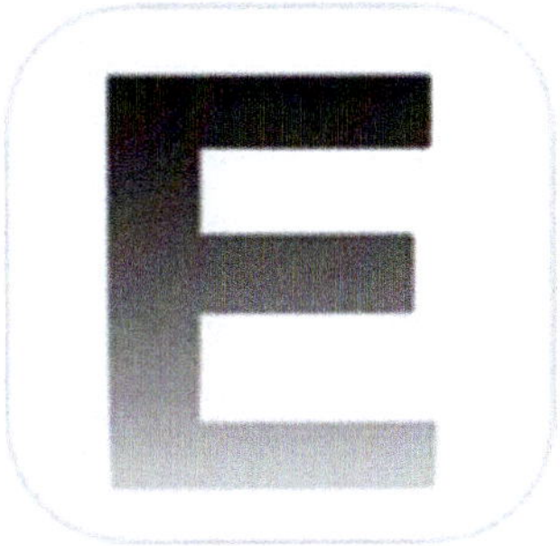

- ***App Screenshots***:

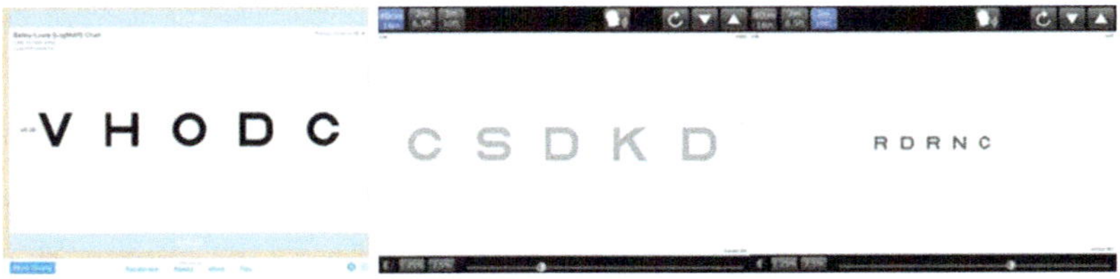

- ***Features***:
  In this Variable Contrast Sensitivity Chart, both the visual acuity and contrast sensitivity may be detected. Contrast testing is done in a logarithmic progression. This progression results in every three rows representing a halving or doubling of visual acuity levels. This allows for better interpretation of the significance of noted visual acuity changes because a three-line difference in the higher acuity ranges would represent the same degree of change as a three-line difference in the lower acuity ranges. Additionally, the separation between optotypes between rows of optotypes has been standardized to be proportional to the size of the optotypes. This results in wider spacing in the lower visual acuity levels and smaller spacing in the higher visual acuity levels.
  Logically, iPad Contrast Sensitivity Eye Charts are superior to the conventional eye charts test because unlike conventional charts the iPad Contrast Sensitivity Eye Charts can measure visual acuity at 100% contrast (the highest contrast) to 1.25% contrast (the lowest contrast). Visual acuity can also be tested at three different distances, 40 cm (16 in.), 2 m (6.5 ft) and 3 m (10 ft), whereas most conventional eye charts can be used only at one distance.

QR Scanning Codes for the App

2. ***Contrast Sensitivity Test***
   - ***Platforms***: Android
   - ***App Creator***: healthcare4mobile
   - ***Version***: 2.0
   - ***App Size***: 9.4 MB
   - ***App Icon***:

   - ***App Screenshots***:

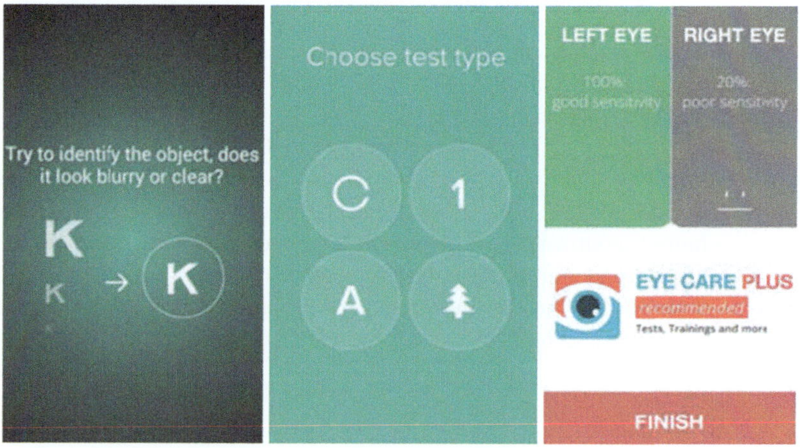

- ***Features***:
  Like the previous app, this app also checks for both visual acuity and contrast sensitivity.

  QR Scanning Codes for the App

3. ***Contrast Sensitivity Function***
   - ***Platforms***: iPhone, iPad
   - ***App Creator***: KyberVision
   - ***Version***: 1.1
   - ***App Size***: 29.8 MB
   - ***App Icon***:

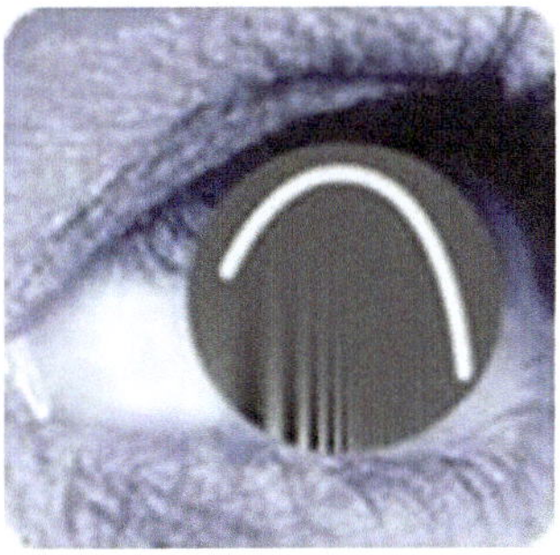

   - ***App Screenshots***:

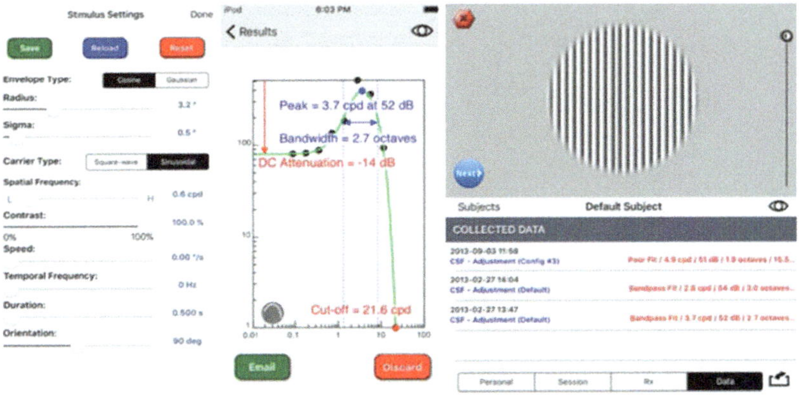

- ***Features***:
  Contrast thresholds are measured by adjusting a contrast slider until the stimulus is barely visible. This process is repeated several times for a range of spatial frequencies. A full contrast sensitivity function (CSF) can then be obtained and fitted with a standard model to derive the descriptive parameters of the CSF: peak frequency, peak sensitivity, bandwidth, cut-off frequency and DC attenuation. The app allows for customizable visual stimuli such as grating, Gabor, static or drifting and multiple stimulus configurations.

  QR Scanning Codes for the App

F. **Apps for Physician Training**

1. ***Eye Handbook***
   - ***Platforms***: iOS (iPhone, iPad, iPod Touch) and Android
   - ***App Creator***: Cloud Nine Development LLC
   - ***Version***: 6.21
   - ***App Size***: 61.3 MB(iOS), 27 MB(Android)
   - ***App Icon***:

- ***App Screenshot***:

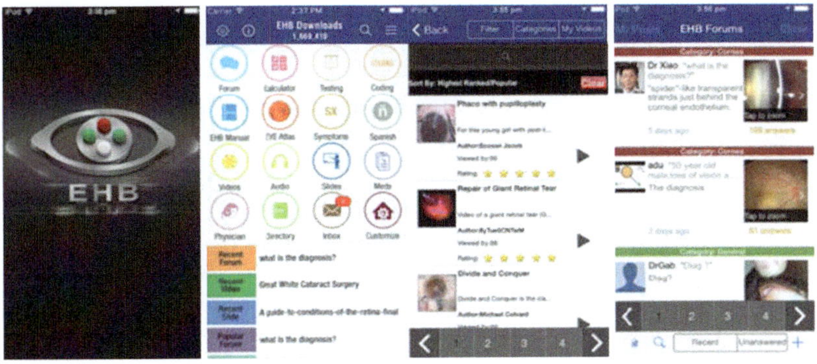

- ***Features***:
  Eye Handbook is one of the most comprehensive diagnostic and treatment reference apps for eye care professionals. Some of the features included are calculators, ICD-9 and ICD-10 coding, eye atlas, differential diagnosis, eponyms and journals. This app is available for free, but it also includes in-app purchases.

  QR Scanning Code for the App

  iOS Android

2. ***EyesHaveIt***
   - ***Platforms***: iOS (iPhone, iPad, iPod Touch)
   - ***App Creator***: The University of Michigan
   - ***Version***: 2.1
   - ***App Size***: 36.8 MB
   - ***App Icon***:

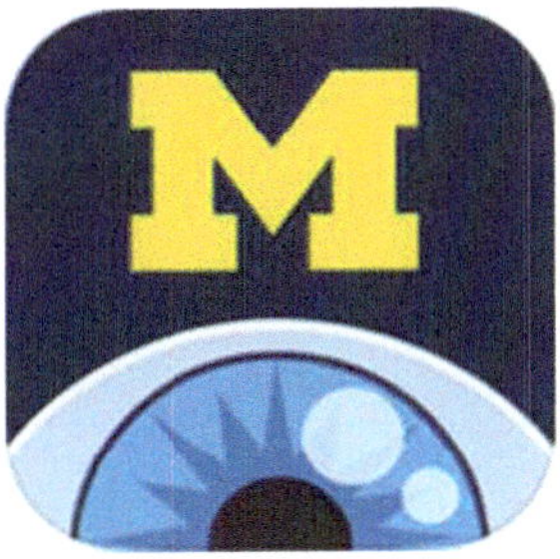

- ***App Screenshots***:

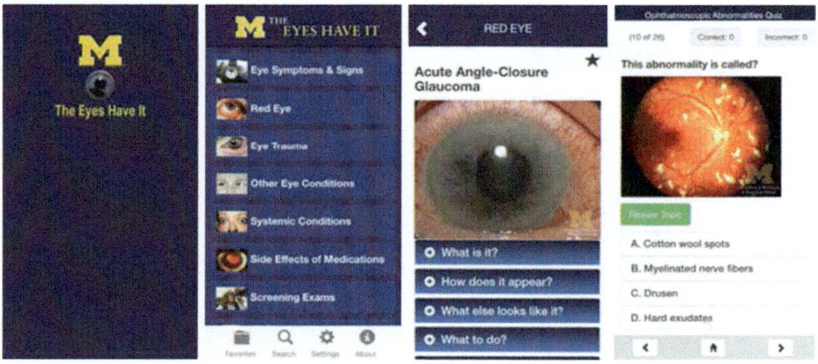

- ***Features***:
  The Eyes Have It (TEHI) app has been developed by University of Michigan ophthalmologist, Dr. Jonathan D. Trobe. The app is intended for medical and optometric students as a learning tool, as well as physicians, optometrists, ophthalmic technicians and other healthcare providers to aid them in diagnosis and management of eye problems.
  The app is a pocket resource with 134 eye conditions, explained with 410 images, more than 40 narrated animations and videos, 6 screening examination videos and an eye anatomy review section. There is also a quiz of multiple-choice questions, allowing students and residents to test themselves on their knowledge of eye conditions and their management.

  QR Scanning Code for the App

3. ***Ophthalmology Training***
   - ***Platforms***: Android, iOS
   - ***App Creator***: Polwarth Medical Ltd.
   - ***Version***: 1.0
   - ***App Size***: 18 MB (Android), 22.9 MB (iOS)

- ***App Icon***:

- ***App Screenshots***:

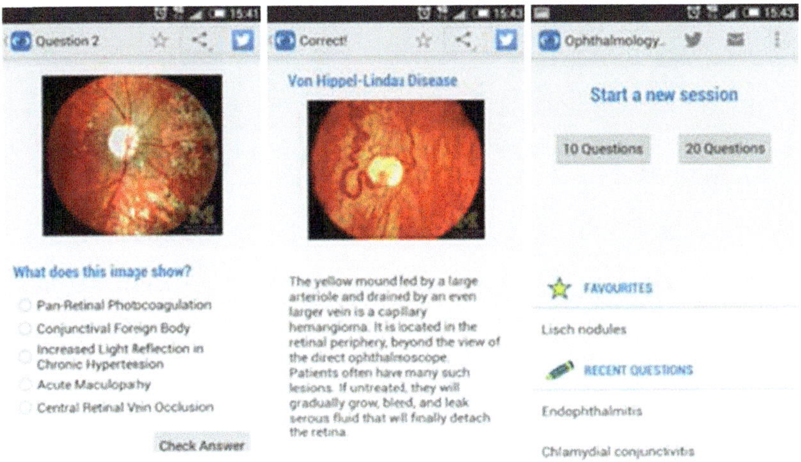

- ***Features***:
  This educational quiz app is designed for medical students, ophthalmologists, opticians, optometrist and healthcare professionals. It covers not only common but also rarer signs and symptoms of principle ophthalmic pathologies, ophthalmic trauma, adverse effects of systemic medications and manifestations of congenital, hereditary and acquired systemic diseases.

  QR Scanning Code for the App

  Android iOS

Social Networking

A. ***Web Resources***

1. ***EyeGuru.org***

   This website has been developed by two ophthalmology residents and a medical student for beginning ophthalmology residents. The site is not suitable at the present time as an in-depth resource for established ophthalmologists. The website features 12 organized courses, which discuss common diseases and examinations techniques. The site offers high-resolution images of the common pathologies and offers practical tips to survive residency.

   Website Screenshot:

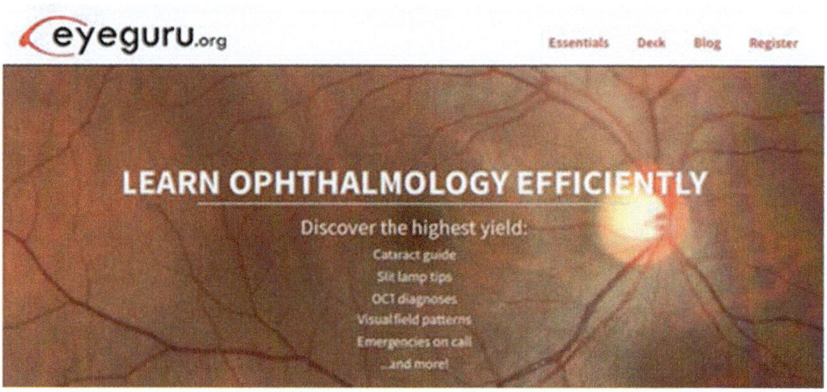

   Site URL: ***http://eyeguru.org***

2. ***University of Iowa's Eye Rounds***

   This webpage is one of the largest online repositories of case presentations and clinical atlases. Both common and rare cases are discussed, and the content is reviewed by an editorial board. There are links to gonioscopy.org, which has a wide variety of gonio images and videos of gonioscopy. There are tutorials about clinical skills, detailed case discussions and literature reviews.

Website Screenshot:

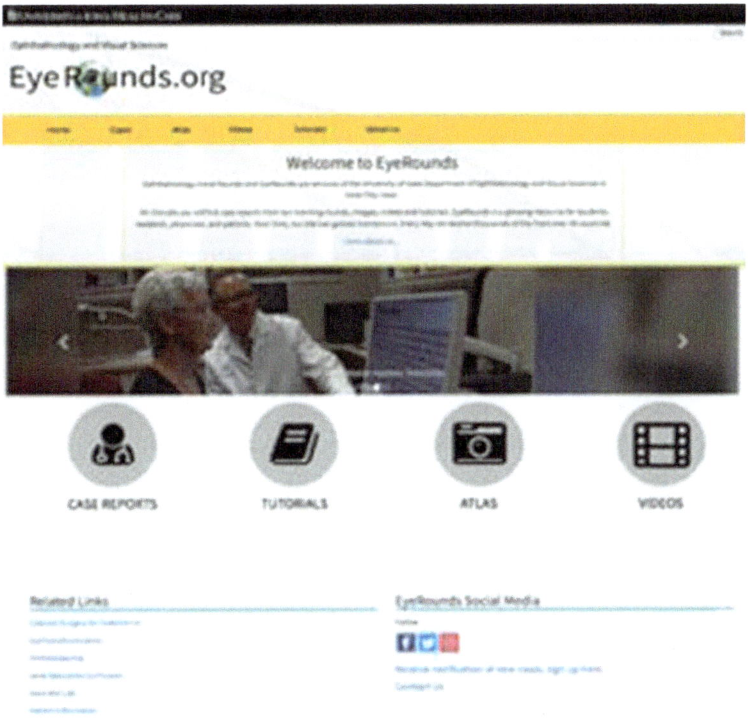

Site URL: ***http://www.eyerounds.org***

3. ***Columbia University's Digital Reference of Ophthalmology***
   This digital atlas contains captioned images of many common ophthalmologic diseases, specific findings and a few case presentations. This is a good resource for budding ophthalmologists for training their mind for pattern recognition.

   Website Screenshots:

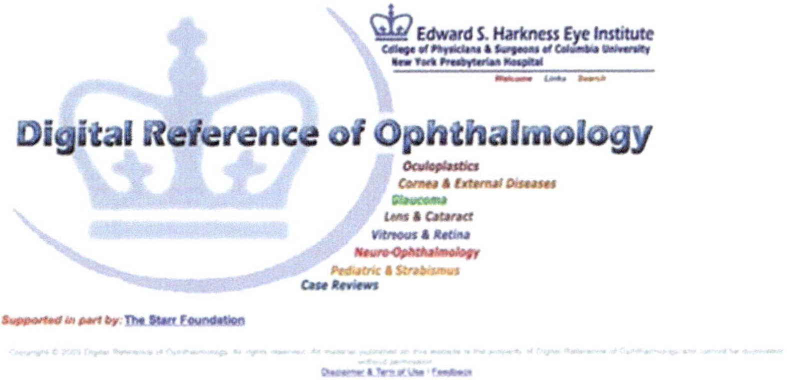

Site URL: ***http://dro.hs.columbia.edu***

4. ***Atlas of Ophthalmology***
   This web atlas has a wide array of pertinent images of various ocular conditions and diagnostic tests organized subspeciality wise. This web resource is endorsed by the International Council of Ophthalmology.

   Website Screenshots:

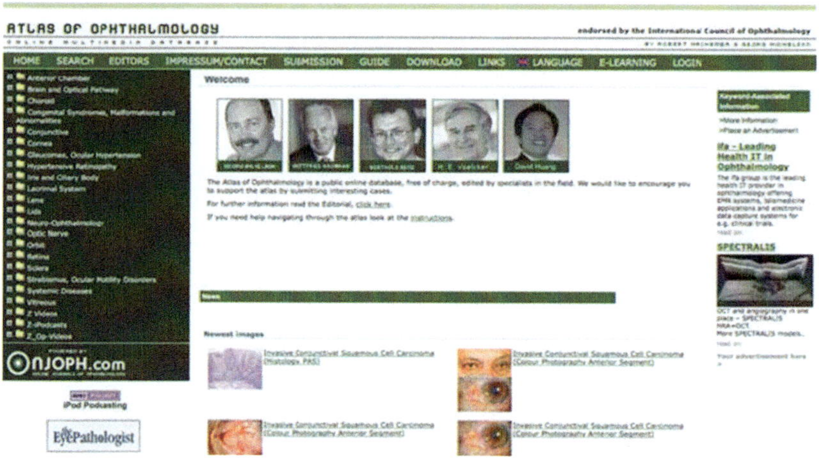

   Site URL: ***https://www.atlasophthalmology.net***

5. ***Ophthobook.com (Part of the Root Eye Network)***
   This webpage offers a free e-book, which is a good and fun learning resource for the residents in ophthalmology. The webpage also offers a terminology dictionary and a video atlas.

   Website Screenshot:

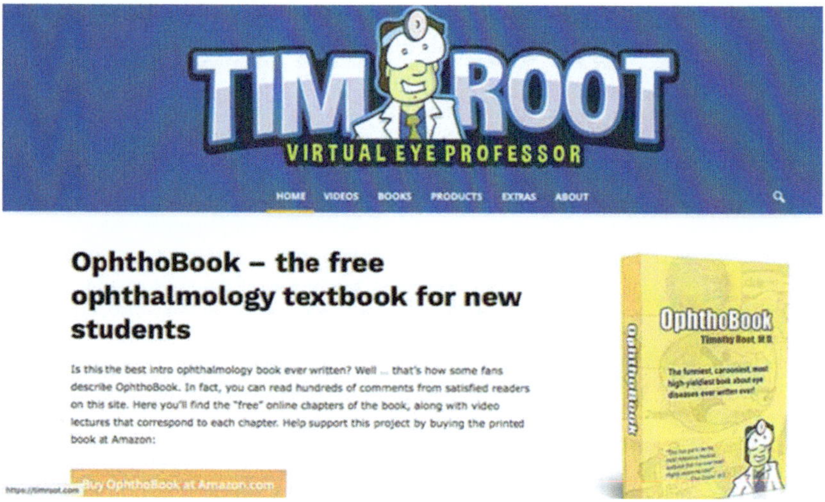

   Site URL: ***https://timroot.com/ophthobook***

B. ***Facebook Pages***

Facebook is no longer just a social tool but a very important educational tool. It's a good tool to share knowledge beyond the boundaries of one's institution and also helps people to collaborate on projects. Additionally, it adds a personal dimension to professional relations. Here are some of the Facebook pages that would interest an ophthalmology resident or fellow.

S. no	Page icon	Page name	Description	QR code
1.	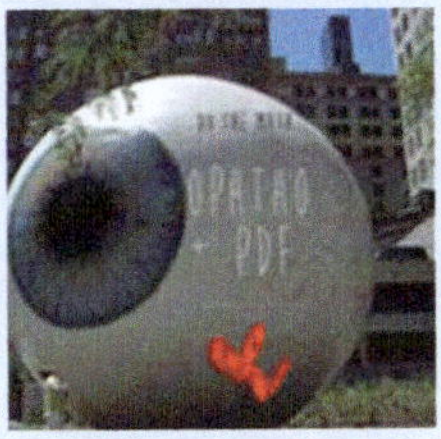	Ophthalmology PDF @pdfophtho	Shares free PDFs of most ophthalmology books	
2.	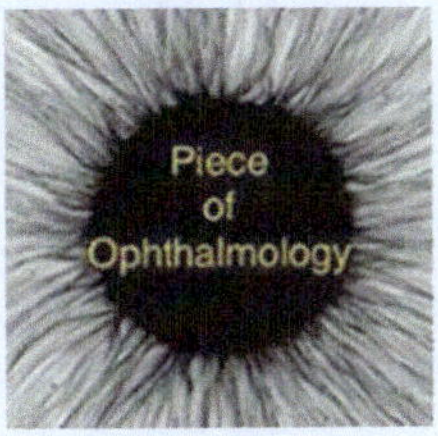	Piece of ophthalmology @PieceOf Ophthalmology	Shares potpourri of information in the form of videos, latest research, excerpts from books and clinical photographs	
3.	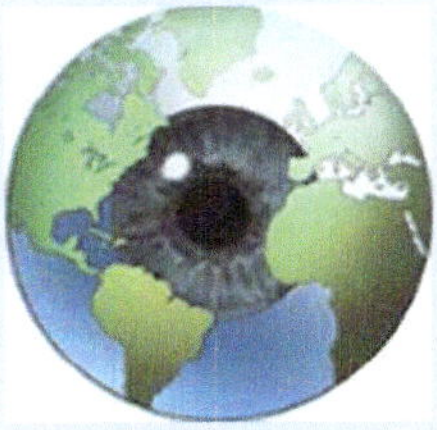	EyeRounds.org @eyerounds	Shares cases from grand rounds at ophthalmology department at University of Iowa, tutorials, atlas and videos	
4.	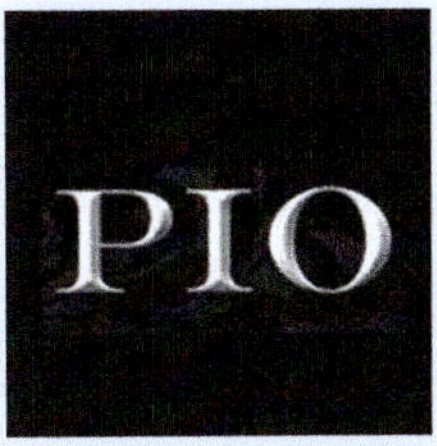	Pearls in Ophthalmology @Pearls InOphtha lmology	The page helps young ophthalmologists to foster exchange of ideas and soft skills such as networking	

S. no	Page icon	Page name	Description	QR code
5.		Ophthalmology Buzzwords @OphthalmologyBuzzwords	Provides high-yield review for the OKAP and boards for ophthalmology residents	
6.		Atlas in Ophthalmology @ophthalmologyatlas	Shares ophthalmic images and cases	
7.		Ophthalmology Pearls @OphthalmologyPearls	This page is affiliated with ophthalmology quiz. Shares clinical photographs, audios and videos	

So, all the smartphone savvy ophthalmologists can now leverage the power of the smart device and squeeze their inventory in their palm.

References

1. Pathipati AS, Wood EH, Lam CK, Sáles CS, Moshfeghi DM. Visual acuity measured with a smartphone app is more accurate than Snellen testing by emergency department providers. Graefes Arch Clin Exp Ophthalmol. 2016;254(6):1175–80.
2. Zhang ZT, Zhang SC, Huang XG, et al. A pilot trial of the iPad tablet computer as a portable device for visual acuity testing. J Telemed Telecare. 2013;19(1):55–9.
3. Tofigh S, Shortridge E, Elkeeb A, Godley BF. Effectiveness of a smartphone application for testing near visual acuity. Eye (Lond). 2015;29(11):1464–8.

4. Bastawrous A, Rono H, Livingstone IA, et al. The development and validation of a smartphone visual acuity test (peek acuity) for clinical practice and community-based fieldwork. JAMA Ophthalmol. 2015;133(8):930–7.
5. Campbell TG, Lehn A, Blum S, Airey C, Brown H. iPad colour vision apps for dyschromatopsia screening. J Clin Neurosci. 2016;29:92–4.
6. Sorkin N, Rosenblatt A, Cohen E, Ohana O, Stolovitch C, Dotan G. Comparison of Ishihara Booklet with color vision smartphone applications. Optom Vis Sci. 2016;93(7):667–72.

Apps and Social Networking Pages for Refractive and Lens-Related Disorders

3

Technical advances in phacoemulsification have not only improved the safety and predictability of cataract surgery but also raised the expectations of both patients and surgeons. All cataract surgeons focus on meeting the individual refractive goal for each patient. Implantation of premium intraocular lenses (IOLs), such as toric IOLs, multifocal IOLs and multifocal toric IOLs, is the fastest-growing segment of refractive eye care. The use of premium IOLs has enhanced the need for precise details of keratometry and topography, for optimum refractive results. Many smartphone apps are contributing towards this goal.

Applications

Apps in this chapter will be discussed under the following heads:

A. Apps for routine intraocular lens power calculation
B. Apps for astigmatism and toric intraocular lenses
C. Educational apps for physicians and patients

A. **Apps for Routine Intraocular Lens Power Calculation**
   1. ***IOL Calculator***
      - ***Platforms***: iPhone and iPad
      - ***App Creator***: Columbia University
      - ***Version***: 1.0
      - ***App Size***: 117.9KB

P. Ichhpujani, S. Thakur, *Smart Resources in Ophthalmology*, Current Practices in Ophthalmology, https://doi.org/10.1007/978-981-13-0140-7_3

- ***App Icon***:

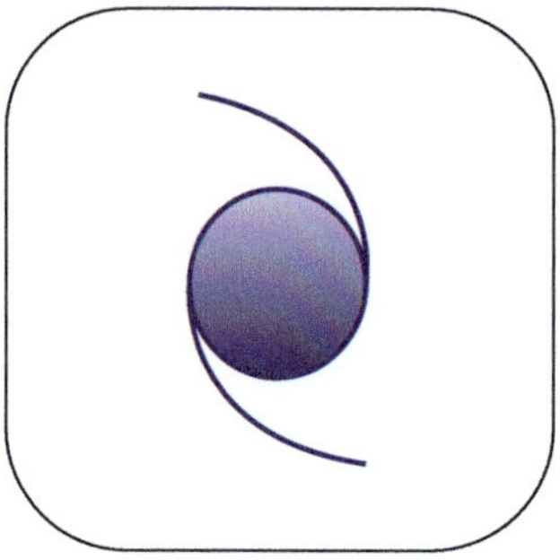

- ***App Screenshots***:

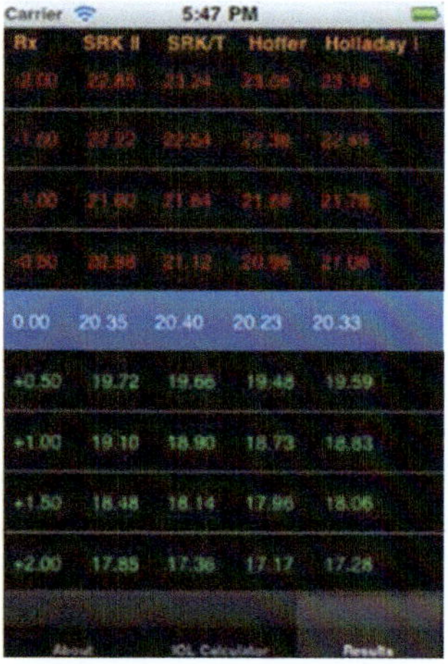

- ***Features***:
  This app helps calculate intraocular power for cataract surgery.

- ***QR Scanning Code of the App***

2. ***IOL Power Calculator (Easy and Accurate)***
   - ***Platforms***: Android
   - ***App Creator***: abhiWorld
   - ***Version***: 1.0
   - ***App Size***: 1.3MB
   - ***App Icon***:

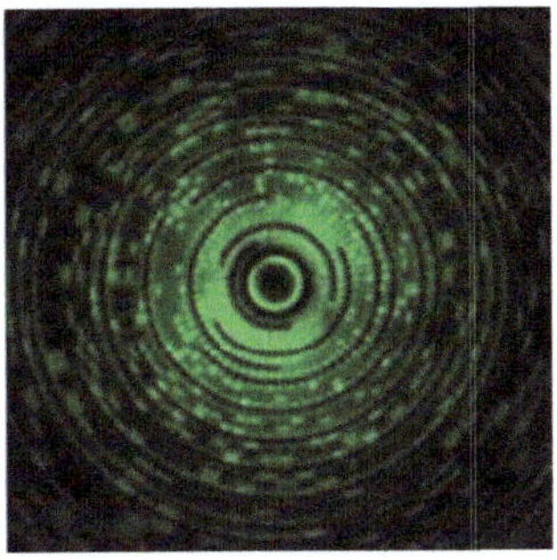

   - ***App Screenshot***:

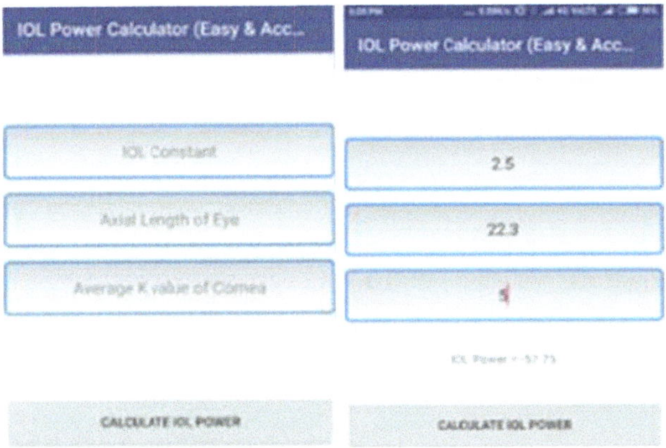

   - ***Features***:
     This app uses a SRK II IOL power calculator with IOL power modification due to axial length variations.

     QR Scanning Code for the App

3. ***BESSt 2***
   - ***Platforms***: iPhone, iPad, iPod Touch
   - ***App Creator***: EB Eye Limited
   - ***Version***: 1.8.1
   - ***App Size***: 14.4 MB
   - ***App Icon***:

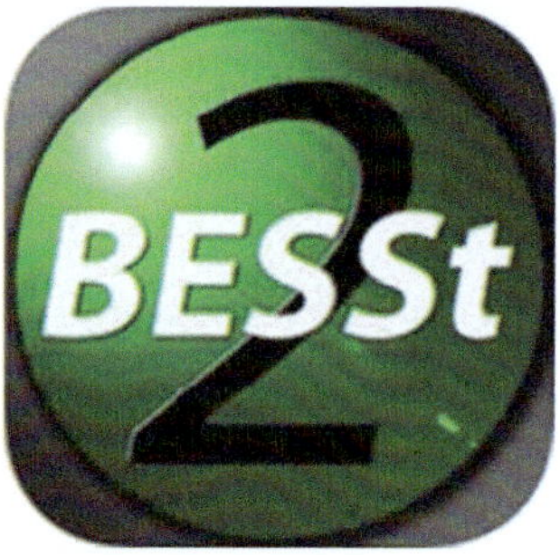

   - ***App Screenshots***:

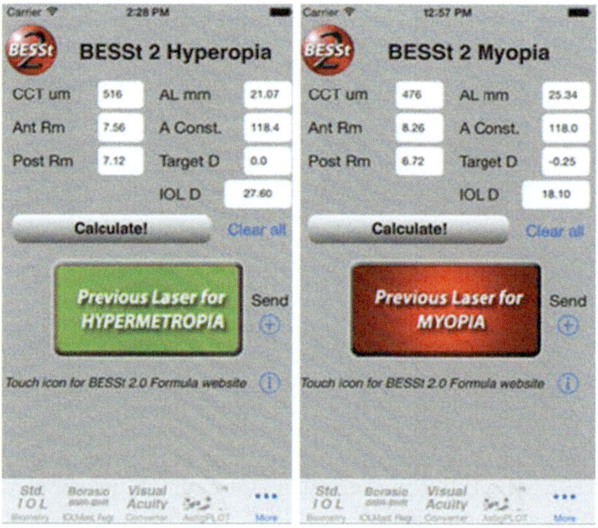

   - ***Features***:
     This app can either be downloaded as a stand-alone app or its features can be used via the Eye Pro 13 app. The app has the latest version of BESSt formula which helps in accurate estimation of IOL power in the eyes that have undergone laser refractive surgery for either hypermetropia or myopia. BESSt 2.0 does not require any pre-refractive surgery information; it only requires Pentacam™ measurements. When using BESSt 2.0 formula, 0 (zero) must be entered in the Sph Aber field. For the surgeons whose Pentacam™ unit does not support Zernike wavefront analysis, BESSt 1.0 formula can be used.

QR Scanning Code for the App

4. ***Cataract and Refractive Imaging Platform***
   - ***Platform***: iPhone, iPad
   - ***App Creator***: *Heidelberg Engineering GmbH*
   - ***Version***: 1.0
   - ***App Size***: 32.5 MB
   - ***App Icon***:

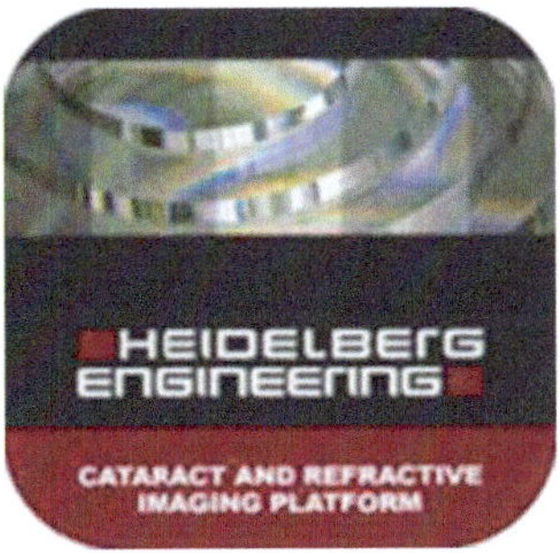

   - ***App Screenshots***:

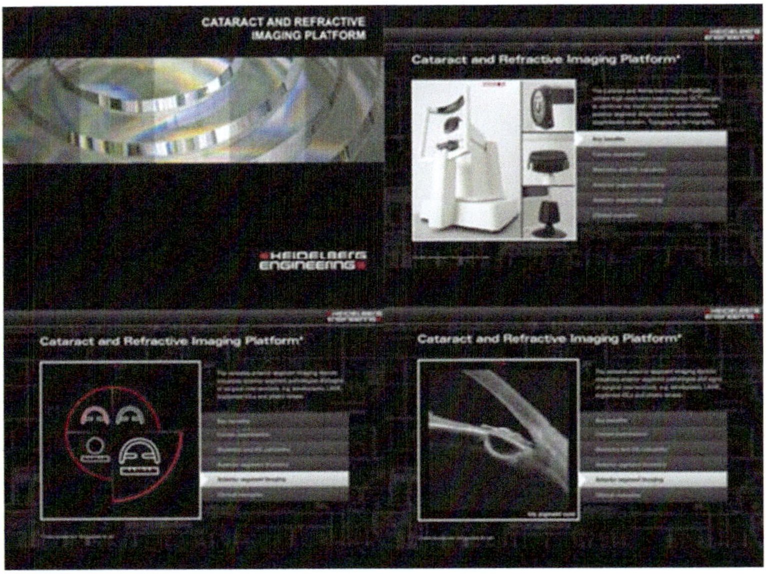

- ***Features***:
  This platform utilizes high-resolution swept-source OCT images to combine the important examinations for anterior segment diagnostics in a modular system. Topography, tomography, anterior segment biometry and axial length data are available in a single workflow efficient platform.

  QR Scanning Code for the App

B. **Apps for Astigmatism and Toric Intraocular Lenses**
Astigmatism following cataract surgery has two components: preoperative, which is intrinsic to the patient, and surgically induced astigmatism (SIA), which is determined by the surgeon's phacoemulsification technique and the type of incision used. It is calculated by comparing pre- and postoperative keratometry values with vector or polar analysis. These calculations have been made easy by several smartphone apps, few of which are enlisted in this section.

1. ***Eye Vectors-Astigmatism Analysis***
   - ***Platforms***: iOS (iPhone and iPad), ($2.99)
   - ***App Creator***: Evandro Souza© Cambui Labs®
   - ***Version***: 5.0
   - ***App Size***: 2.3 MB
   - ***App Icon***:

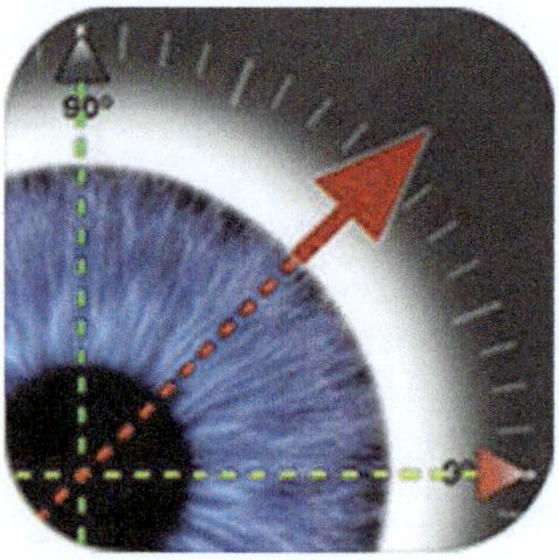

- ***App Screenshots***:

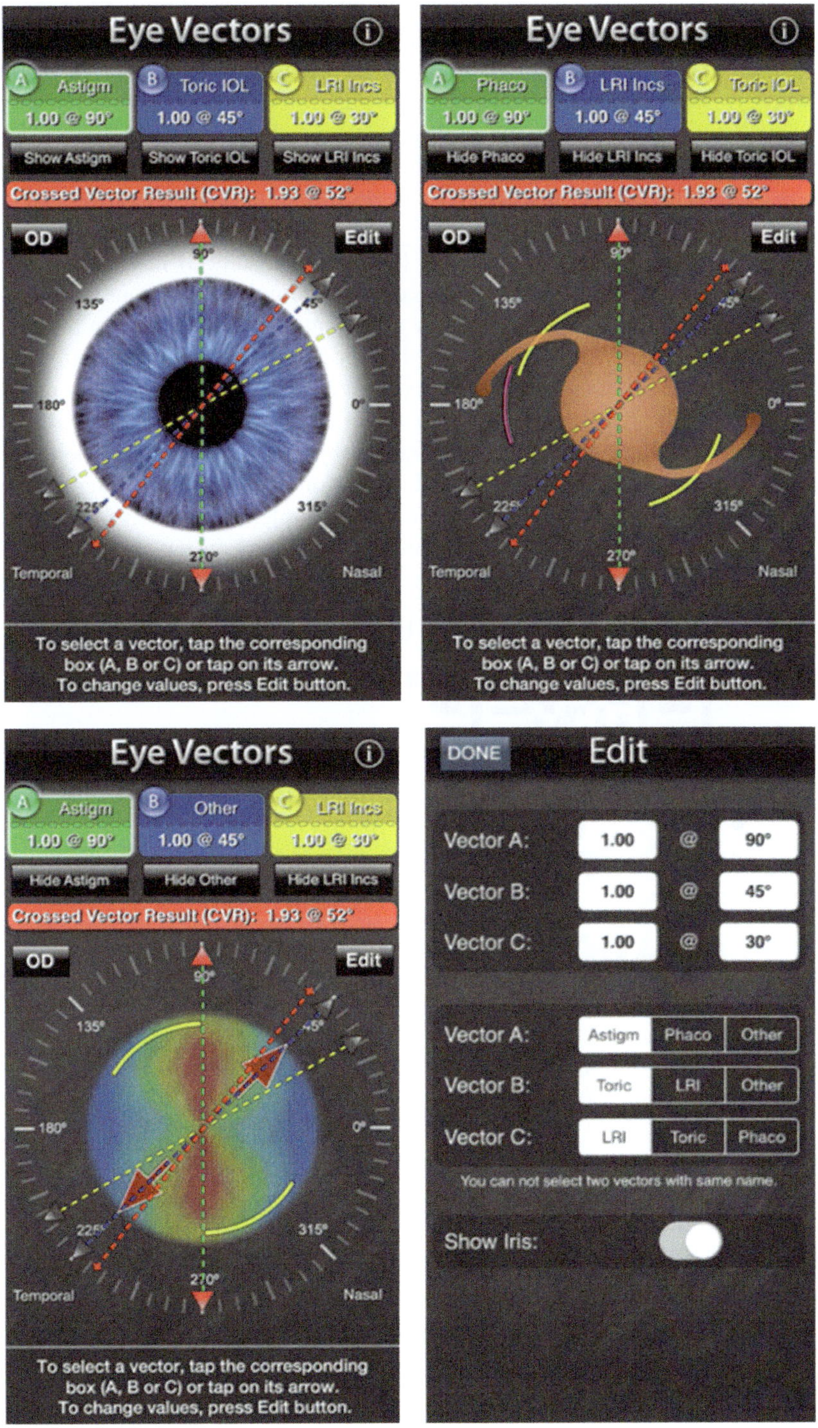

- ***Features***:

  These days cataract surgery is evolving as a refractive surgery, and surgeons attempt to use intraocular lenses or limbal relaxing incisions (LRI) or both, to negate pre-existing astigmatism. This app does the vector analysis and shows the resulting two or three forces vectors when projected on the cornea. This app helps to know the final outcome by calculating the intersection of forces of intrinsic astigmatism and additional induced overlapping force (either by phacoemulsification, Toric IOL or LRI).

  There are three vectors (named A, B and C) that can be moved and changed. A vector is selected by tapping the corresponding colour box or touching the tip of its arrow. User can align each vector in the corresponding desired axis by moving his/her finger. The vectors A (green), B (blue) and C (yellow) are the forces, and red is the final cross vector result (CVR). The values induced by each vector or its name can be changed by using the EDIT. If an examiner needs to analyse only two vectors, then they need to enter value 0 @ 0 for the third vector. The user must enter the final value of induction for each vector. For example, if each LRI induces 1.50 dioptres and two incisions are made, 3.00 dioptres is entered in the corresponding vector.

  QR Scanning Code of the App

2. ***Axis Toric Calculator***
   - ***Platforms***: Android
   - ***App Creator***: Omni Lens Pvt. Ltd.
   - ***Version***: 1.0.2
   - ***App Size***: 7.1 MB

- ***App Icon***:

- ***App Screenshots***:

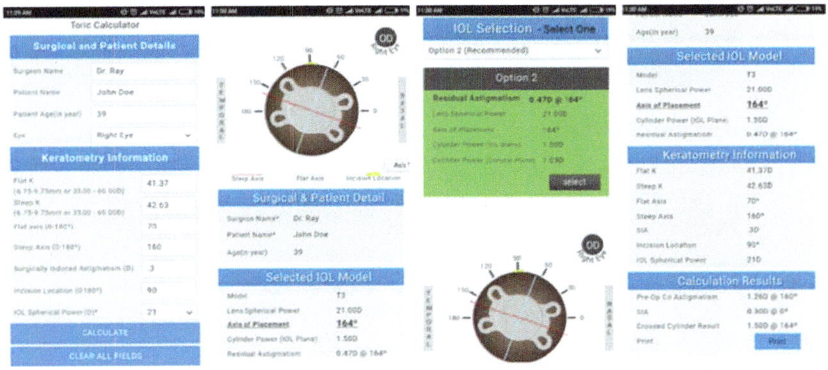

- ***Features***:

This calculator is used as an adjunct with comprehensive ocular examination and appropriate diagnostic tests pre-cataract surgery.

The toric tool provides a starting point for the toric IOL selection and modification. The final prescription must be determined by the surgeon's routine toric lens fitting practices.

QR Scanning Code for the App

3. ***Astig Master***
   - ***Platforms***: iPhone; iPad
   - ***App Creator***: EB Eye Limited
   - ***Version***: 1.7.1
   - ***App Size***: 14.5 MB
   - ***App Icon***:

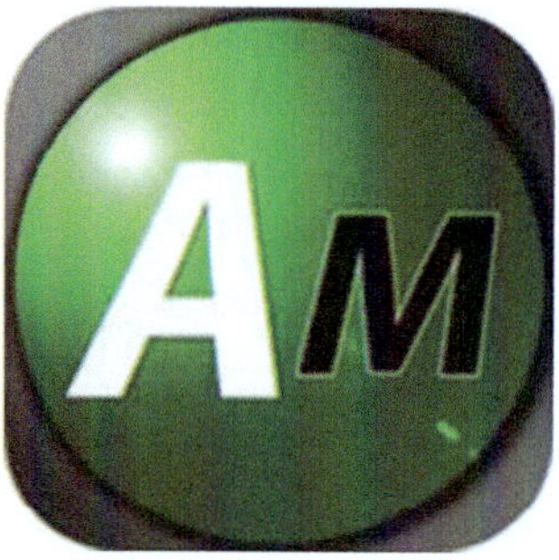

   - ***App Screenshots***:

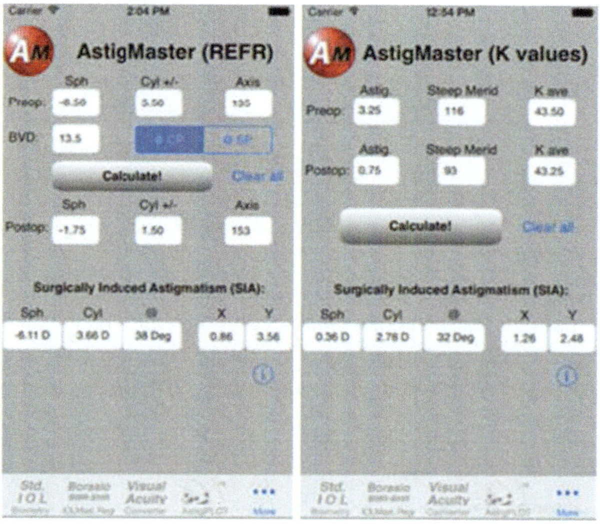

   - ***Features***:
     This app allows an anterior segment surgeon to calculate the surgically induced astigmatism vector.

QR Scanning Code for the App

4. ***AstigPlot***
   - ***Platforms***: iPhone, iPad, iPod Touch
   - ***App Creator***: EB Eye Limited
   - ***Version***: 1.4
   - ***App Size***: 15.1 MB
   - ***App Icon***:

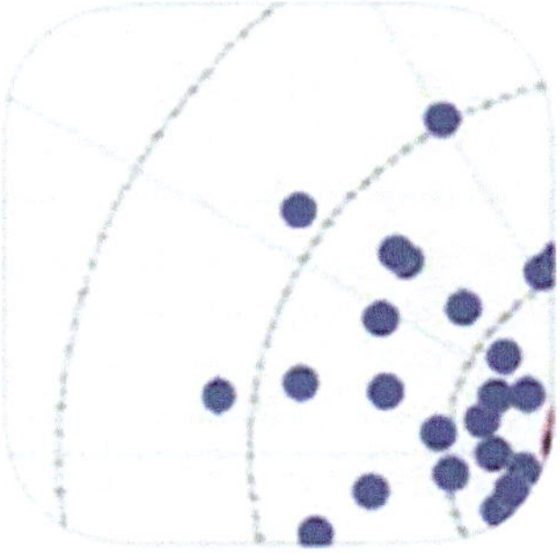

   - ***App Screenshots***:

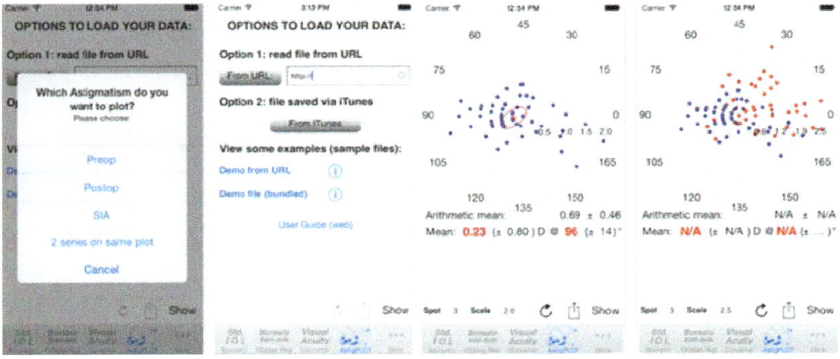

   - ***Features***

The application plots pre-op and post-op astigmatism and aggregates astigmatism, SIA and mean astigmatism. It also calculates the standard deviation of the mean astigmatism and the surgeon's SIA. The SIA is not only shown in terms of sphere, cylinder along with its axis but also as the Cartesian (x,y) notation. Cartesian notation is required for calculation of the mean of multiple individual SIAs.

QR Scanning Code for the App

5. ***Eye Pro 2013***
   - ***Platforms***: iPhone, iPad, iPod Touch
   - ***App Creator***: EB Eye Limited
   - ***Version***: 1.5.1
   - ***App Size***: 14.7 MB
   - ***App Icon***:

   - ***App Screenshot***:

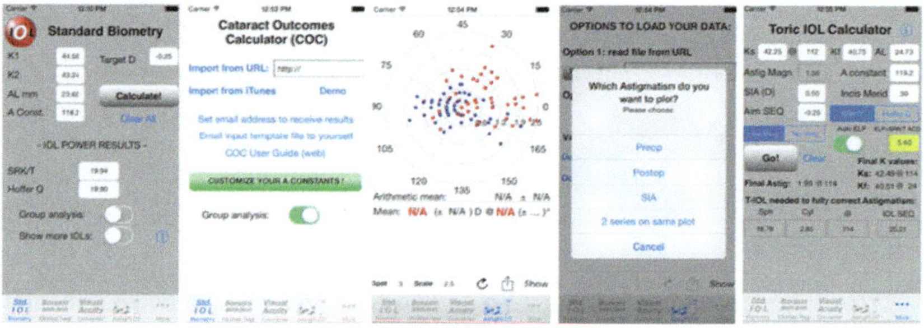

- ***Features***:

  This app is a comprehensive app for a cataract surgery as it offers a wide array of calculators and analysis. The app has the following features:
  - Visual acuity converter (between LogMar, Snellen and Decimal notation)
  - Standard biometry
  - Phaco outcomes calculator (mean biometry error and SD)
  - Biometry post-laser refractive surgery
  - SIA calculator for single cases and group of the eyes
  - Corneal-spectacle plane converter
  - Cartesian-polar notation converter
  - Astigmatism correction reduction calculator, which predicts the final astigmatism following incision misplacement or toric IOL misalignment
  - Toric IOL calculators

  QR Scanning Code for the App

6. ***LRI Calc-Limbal Relaxing Incisions***
   - ***Platforms***: iPhone, iPad, iPod Touch
   - ***App Creator***: Evandro Souza
   - ***Version***: 2.0
   - ***App Size***: 7.7 MB
   - ***App Icon***:

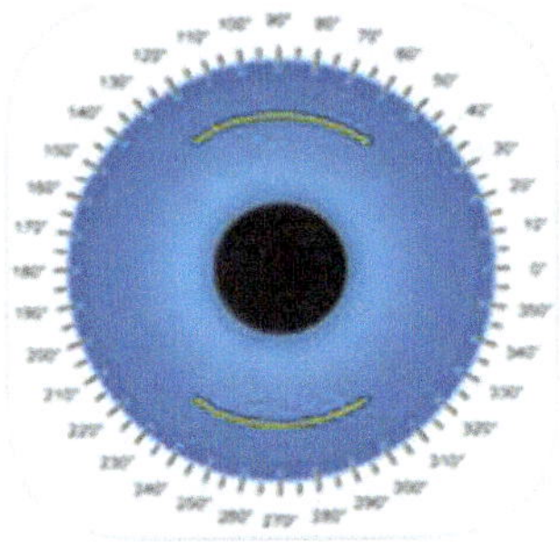

- ***App Screenshots***:

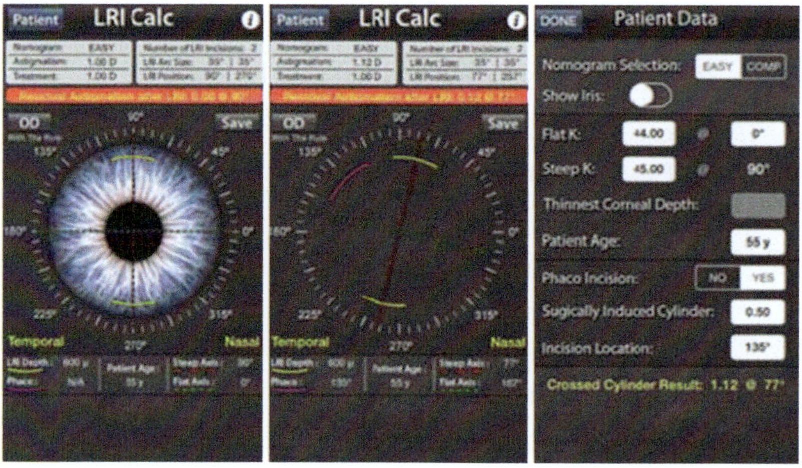

- ***Features***:
  This app helps in preoperative planning for limbal relaxing incisions (LRI) to correct the astigmatism.

  QR Scanning Code for the App

7. ***Toreasy/TorAxis***
   - ***Platforms***: Toreasy (Android), TorAxis(iOS) (English, French)
   - ***App Creator***: Bsoft.fr
   - ***Version***: 2.0.3
   - ***App Size***: 6.8 MB
   - ***App Icon***:

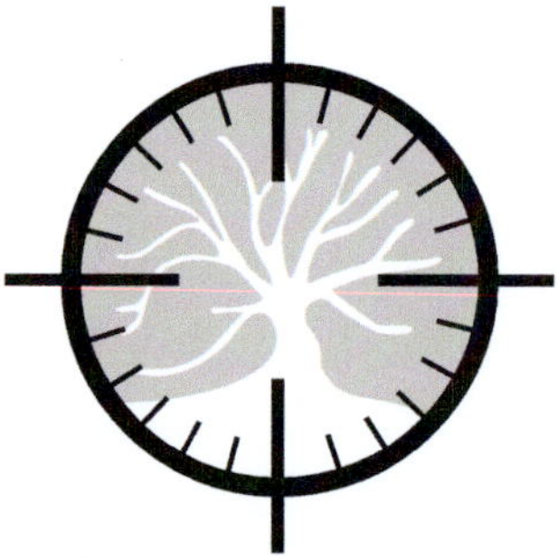

- ***App Screenshot***:

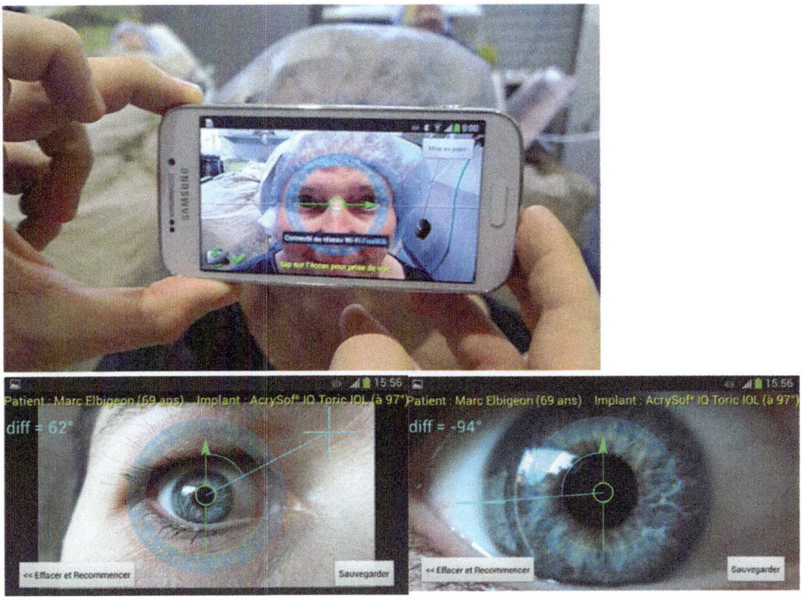

- ***Features***:

  Modern smartphones are equipped with gyroscope and accelerometer sensors in order to track the position of the smartphone and to provide its user with stable and reliable orientation in space.

  Smartphones can therefore, display an artificial horizon line superimposed on the camera view screen, even if they are not held in perfect horizontal or vertical orientation. They can also display a circular reticule, graduated over 360°, to allow location of any pinpoint on the screen with an angular precision of less than 1°.

  Toreasy/TorAxis app is used for toric IOL alignment. It has a trial version and an unlimited version. When using the app, patient's head is positioned so that a virtual horizontal line crosses the pupils of the right and left eyes. Then a snapshot of the eye is taken. Augmented reality azimuth marks, which are continuously realigned using the gyroscope sensors, are then displayed on the visualization screen. The high-definition snapshot of the eye allows the user to zoom in, so that any element such as a blood vessel, pigmentation mark, etc. can be easily located and its exact angle coordinates determined in order to establish a reliable orientation mark. Once the patient is prepped and draped, the desired toric IOL axis orientation can be referenced on the patient's eye during surgery using a Mendez ring or projection technology built into the surgical microscope.

QR Scanning Code of the App

iOS Android

8. ***toriCAM***
   - ***Platforms***: iPhone, iPad, iPod Touch
   - ***App Creator***: Graham Barrett
   - ***Version***: 3.0
   - ***App Size***: 1.9 MB
   - ***App Icon***:

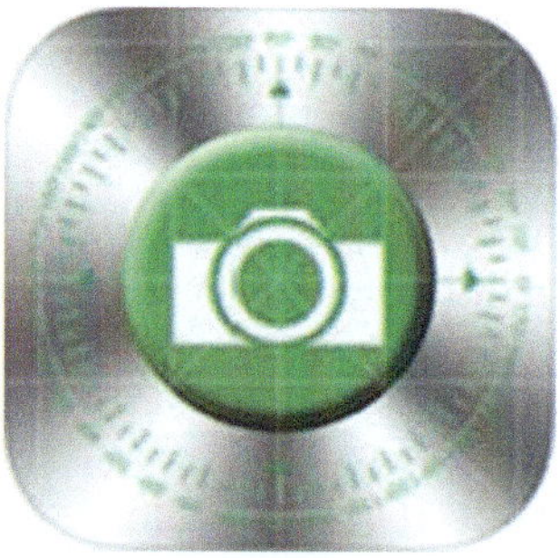

   - ***App Screenshots***:

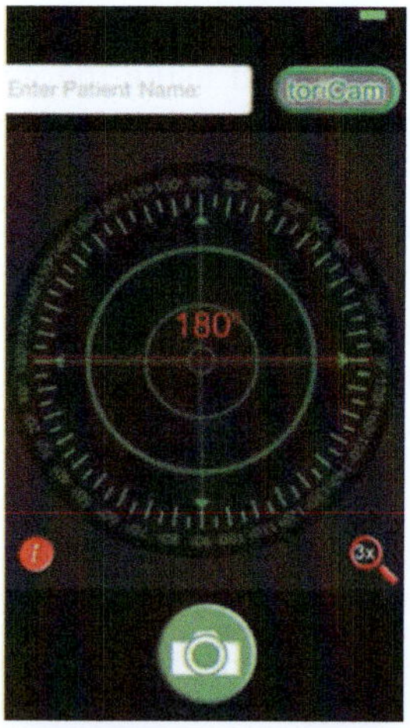

- ***Features***:

  This app helps to determine the axis of corneal limbal marks used as a reference to determine the correct alignment for a toric IOL at the time of surgery. It can also be used to measure the axis of an implanted IOL at the slit lamp postoperatively.

  QR Scanning Code for the App

C. **Educational Apps for Physicians and Patients**

1. ***Lens NAVI***
   - ***Platforms***: iPhone and iPad (English and German)
   - ***App Creator***: Ronald Krueger
   - ***Version***: 1.3
   - ***App Size***: 2.3MB
   - ***App Icon***:

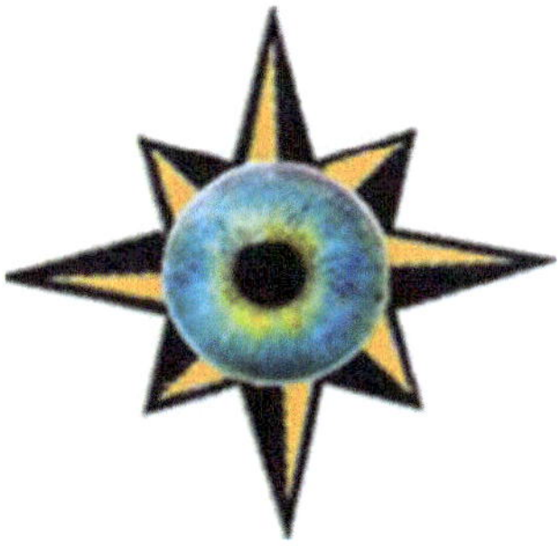

- ***App Screenshots***:

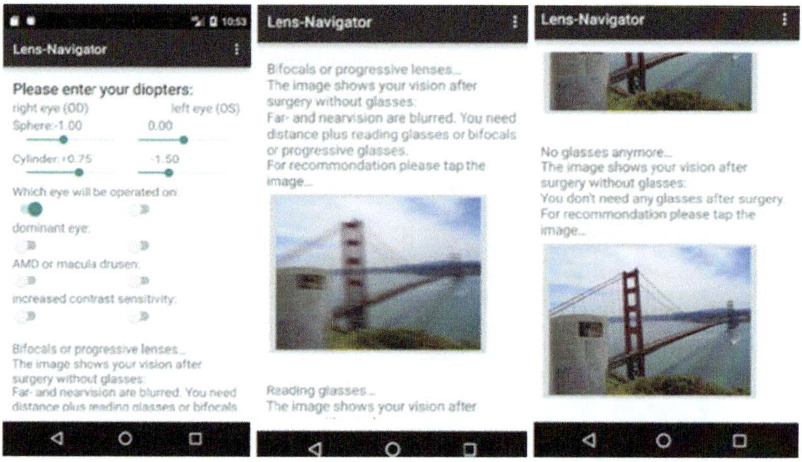

- ***Features***:
  Due to the wide variety of different intraocular lenses (mono-/multifocal, aspheric, toric, blue filter, etc.), the postoperative refractive outcome can be very different for the convenience of the patient: reading glasses only, monovision, etc.

  With this app, the patient has to input his/her dioptres and can add additional information, for example, his/her dominant eye, macular pathology, etc. and the desired outcome (e.g. reduced blurring/haze, improved night vision/contrast sensitivity). After tapping the example picture representing the visual impression he/she wants to achieve, he/she will get information about which intraocular lens will meet his expectations in the right and left eye, respectively, and the outcome. If it is not possible to achieve the desired goals, the patient can discuss the choice of intraocular lens with the ophthalmologist. The app results are reduced refractive surprises and satisfactory refractive outcome.

QR Scanning Code of the App

iOS

Android

2. ***cataractDroid***
   - ***Platforms***: Android
   - ***App Creator***: George YX Kong
   - ***Version***: 1.0
   - ***App Size***: 3.6 MB
   - ***App Icon***:

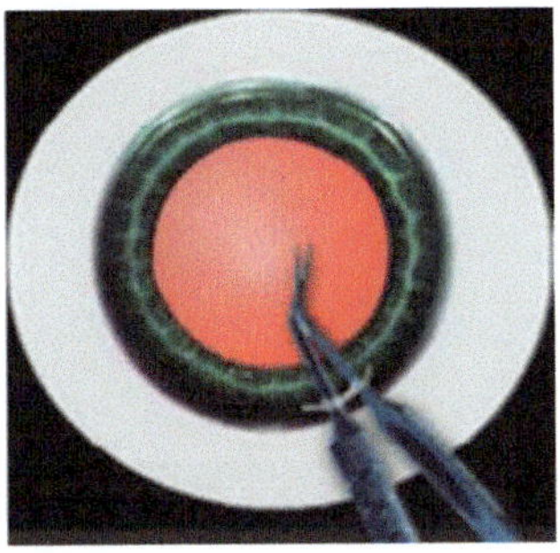

   - ***App screenshots***:

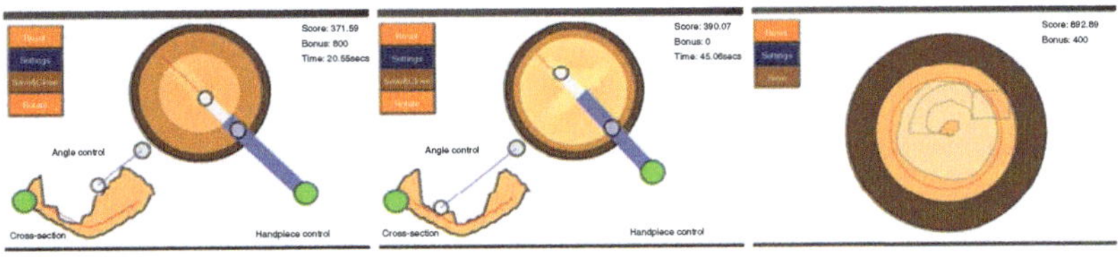

   - ***Features***:

This app is a simulation of capsulorhexis and phacoemulsification. It helps budding surgeons to develop hand-eye coordination. The same app is available on iOS by the name of cataractMobile.

QR Scanning Code for the App

3. ***ESCRS Eurotimes***
   - ***Platform***: iPhone, iPad, Android
   - ***App Creator***: *ESCRS*
   - ***Version***: 4.0.301

- ***App Size***: 31.7MB
- ***App Icon***:

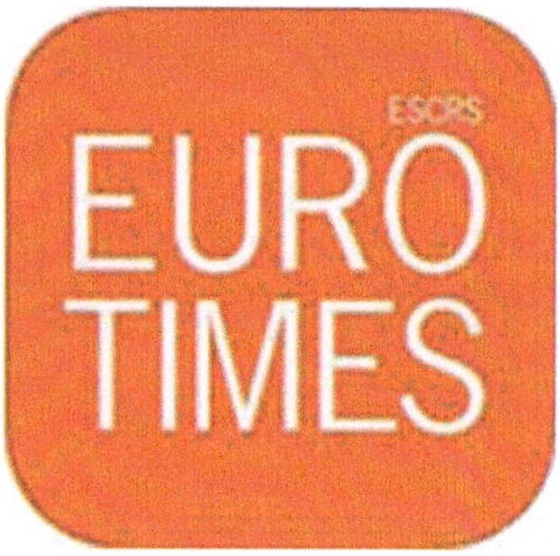

- ***App Screenshot***:

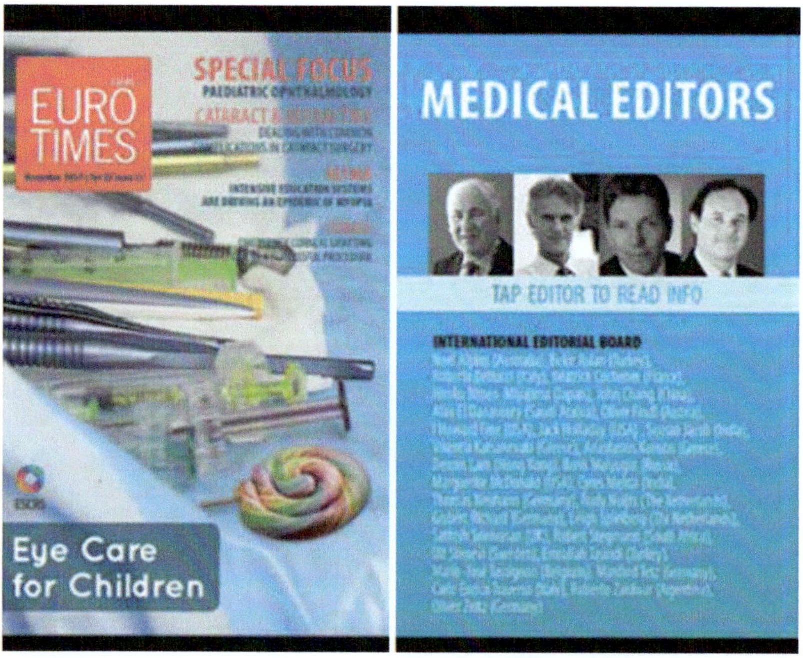

- ***Features***:

  This app updates each issue of the Eurotimes magazine and offers in-depth features on the latest news in ophthalmology with reports and analysis from the major ophthalmic meetings including ASCRS, AAO, ESCRS, WOC, EuCornea, EURETINA and the European Glaucoma Society.

  Additionally, book reviews, travel articles and features on research and young ophthalmologists are also added.

QR Scanning Code for the App

4. ***Journal of Cataract and Refractive Surgery***
   - ***Platform***: iPhone, iPad
   - ***App Creator***: *ESCRS*
   - ***Version***: 7.1.0
   - ***App Size***: 54.9 MB
   - ***App Icon***:

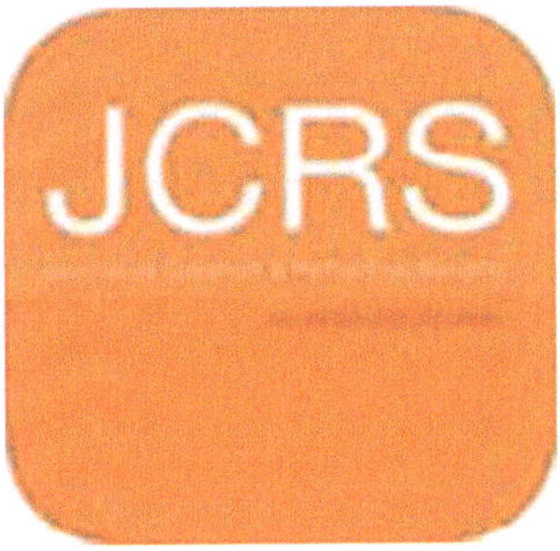

   - ***App Screenshots***:

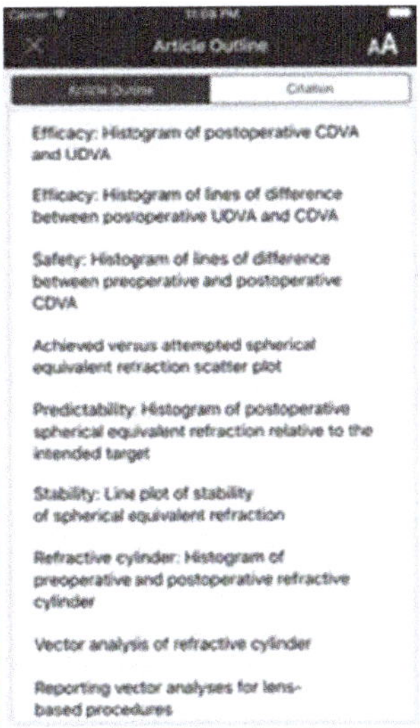

- ***Features***:
  This app helps an ophthalmologist and especially an anterior segment surgeon to stay abreast with latest in the field. The app alerts the user when new issues are available. AudioSlides, Virtual Microscope, 3D Radiological Viewer and 3D Neuroimaging Viewer are the highlights of the app.

  QR Scanning Code for the App

Social Networking

A. ***Websites***

1. ***American Society of Cataract and Refractive Surgery (ASCRS)***

   The official webpage of ASCRS is a good resource for advancing the skills and technique of both budding and established ophthalmic surgeons by providing latest clinical and practice management education. It is a good site for anterior segment relevant published research and regulatory information affecting the practice.

   The website has an online registry for haemorrhagic occlusive retinal vasculitis (HORV). ASCRS has developed a task force to investigate HORV, which is a rare complication of any intraocular procedure (usually cataract surgery) characterized by vision loss occurring 1–6 days after an unremarkable postoperative day 1 examination.

   It also has a toxic anterior segment syndrome (TASS) registry, an ophthalmic product buying guide and a link to the JCRS journal.

   Website Screenshots:

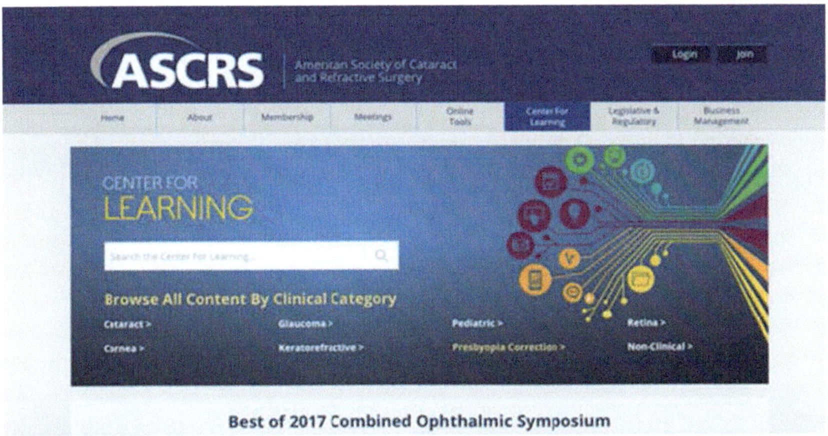

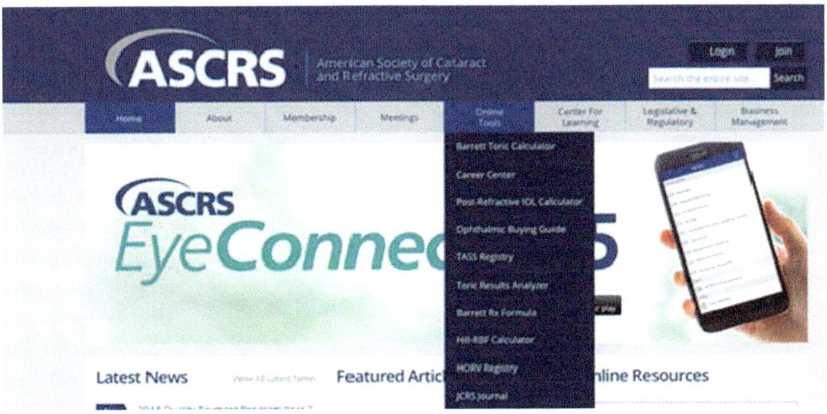

   Site URL: ***http://www.ascrs.org***

2. ***European Society of Cataract and Refractive Surgery (ESCRS)***
   The official webpage of ESCRS. It has an elearning section for its members which offers interactive, accredited elearning content, including surgical videos, diagrams, animations, quizzes and forums. It has also has a separate section for European trainee young ophthalmologists (YO), who can apply for a grant to observe clinical practice in a university setting.

   Website Screenshots:

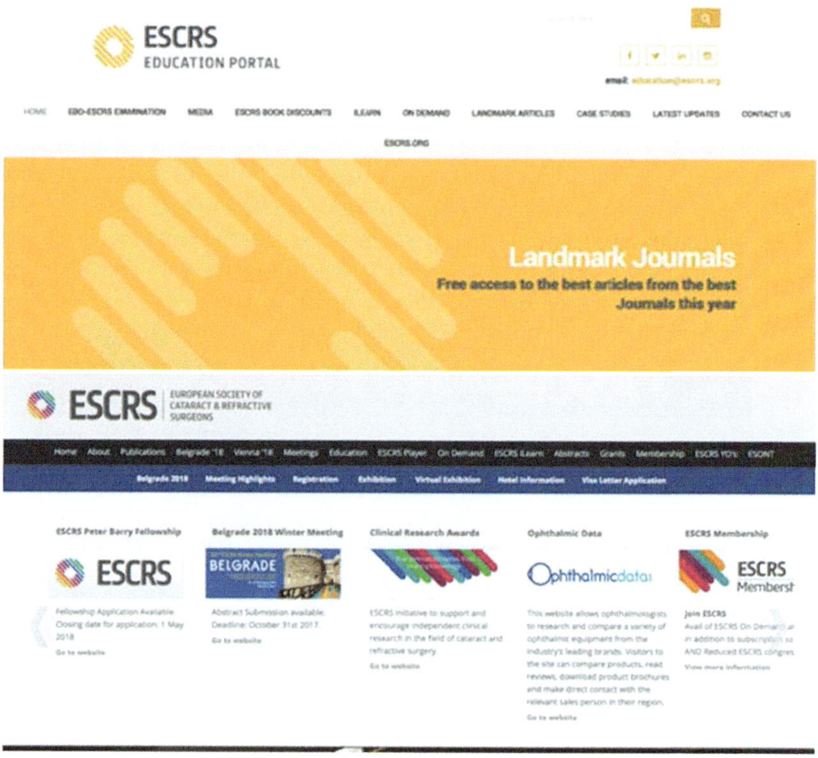

   Site URL: ***http://www.escrs.org***

3. ***Journal of Cataract and Refractive Surgery***
   This is the official webpage of the journal. It is a consolidated portal not just of archives of the journal and its supplements but also has a special section on consultation and surgical techniques.

Website Screenshot:

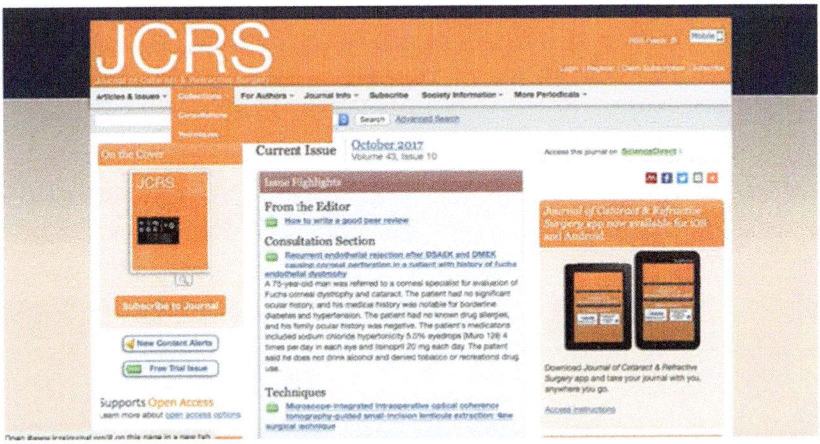

Site URL: ***http://www.jcrsjournal.org***

4. ***International Society of Refractive Surgery (ISRS)***
The International Society of Refractive Surgery (ISRS) is a partner of the American Academy of Ophthalmology (AAO) and is the leading organization for refractive surgeons. The webpage apprises the ophthalmologists of the latest clinical and research developments in refractive, cornea, cataract and lens-based surgery, through its clinical journal, monthly newsletter, innovative educational programmes and meetings around the world.

   The resource centre on the webpage has a concept of K-Card for LASIK patients. Patients preoperative keratometry readings and refraction are noted on the card which is given to LASIK patients, as it is often difficult to track down this critical data later on, when the patient is need of cataract surgery or any additional eye care.

Website Screenshot:

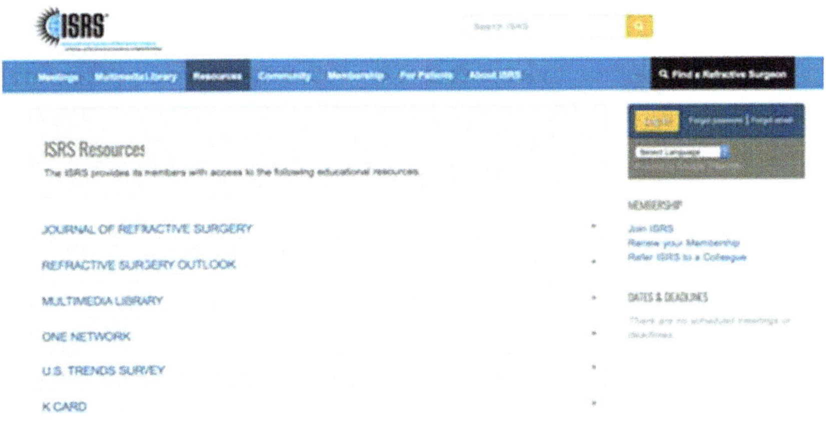

Site URL: ***https://isrs.aao.org***

5. ***Cataract and Refractive Surgery Today (CRST)***
   This webpage is a comprehensive portal for cataract and refractive surgeons. CRST promotes continuing education with the latest surgical approaches and techniques, complications avoidance pearls and management, practice management.

   Website Screenshot:

   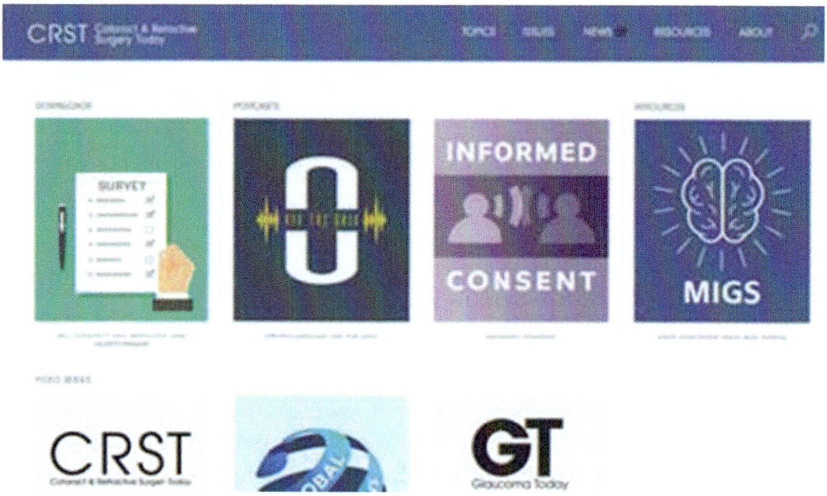

   Site URL: ***https://crstoday.com***

6. ***ASSORT Toric Calculator***
   The USP of this tool is its ability to calculate the most effective implant (sphere and toricity) available from all companies worldwide and compare IOLs based on the target spherocylindrical refraction that is calculated to remain postoperatively .The user need not visit several separate corporate websites.

   The astigmatic effect of the phacoemulsification mainport incision can be dynamically adjusted based on incision placement. A new parameter, corneal topographic astigmatism (CorT total) can also be used for an accurate measure of corneal astigmatism with inclusion of the posterior cornea [1].

Website Screenshot:

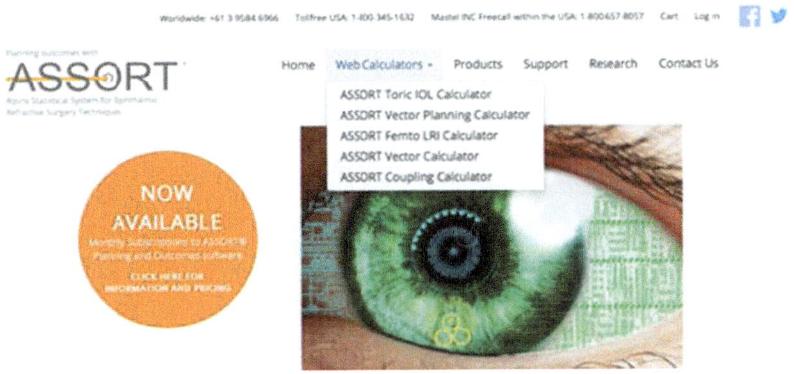

Site URL: *www.assort.com*

7. ***Toric Results Analyser***

This tool helps in dealing with residual astigmatism following toric IOL implantation. For every degree that the orientation of a toric lens differs from the ideal, there is approximately 3.3% decrease in its effectiveness at reducing astigmatism [2].

It also provides information that helps to determine the ideal rotation of the lens to correct residual astigmatism and can provide information for an IOL exchange if a higher or lower toric power is needed. In cases where rotation or exchange would not be useful, laser vision correction is an option.

Website Screenshot:

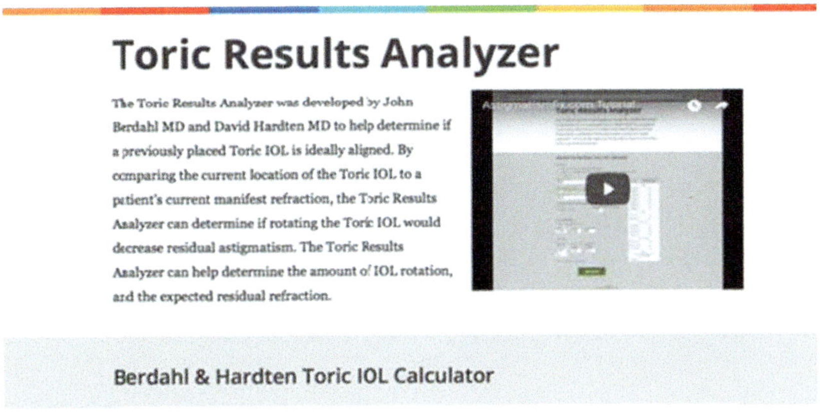

Site URL: ***https://astigmatismfix.com***

B. ***Facebook Pages***

S. no	Page icon	Page name	Description	QR code
Society pages				
1.		International Society of Refractive Surgery @ISRS.org	Platform for anterior segment surgeons to get updates of publishes research, surgical techniques and meetings	
2.		APACRS-Asia Pacific Association of Cataract and Refractive Surgeons @APACRS.secretariat	Shares updates about the society meetings and the latest articles in the magazine, Eyeworld	
3.		The European Society of Cataract and Refractive Surgeons @ESCRS	Shares updates about the society meetings and shares updates from their education portal	
4.		American Society of Cataract and Refractive Surgeons	Official FB page of the society. Shares information about meetings and webinars	

S. no	Page icon	Page name	Description	QR code
Physician information and training				
1.	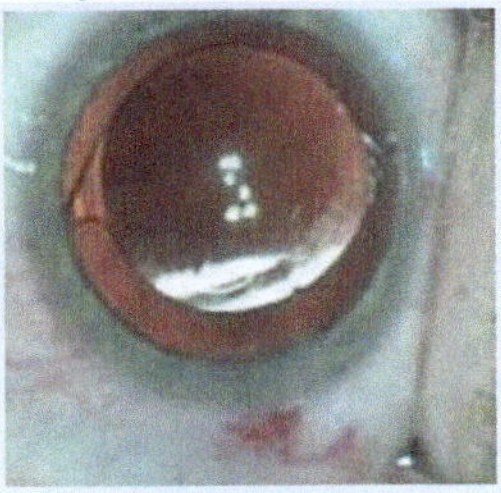	Pearls for Cataract and Refractive Surgeons @ Refractivecataract surgeons	Designed to enhance knowledge for cataract and refractive surgeons with an emphasis on advanced technologies (femtosecond cataract surgery, toric and multifocal IOLs)	
2.	CRST	Cataract and Refractive surgery Today	Delivers cutting-edge information to cataract and refractive surgeons	
3.		Eyetube.net @Eyetube	Shares new surgical techniques to educate ophthalmologists	

C. ***Twitter Handles***

S. no	Handle icon	Handle name	Description	QR code
1.	ASCRS	*ASCRS* @ASCRS tweets	Official account of ASCRS	

S. no	Handle icon	Handle name	Description	QR code
2.		*JCRS* @JCRS	JCRS is the home of anterior segment surgery in ophthalmology, is the official journal of the ASCRS and ESCRS	
3.		*ESCRS* @ESCRSofficial	Official account of the ESCRS, providing society news, educational content and conference coverage from the world of ophthalmology	
4.		*The Ophthalmologist* @OphthoMag	Handle for the magazine; presents groundbreaking innovations in the management of ophthalmic disorders	
5.		*Ophthalmology Times* @OTEurope	Handle for Ophthalmology Times Europe magazine: Offers latest news in cataract, refractive, retina and glaucoma	

All these applications and web resources have empowered the cataract surgeons to achieve the desired refractive outcome, without sitting glued to their desktops for extensive calculations. Happy planning-on the Go!!

References

1. Koch DD, Ali SF, Weikert MP, Shiriyama M, Jenkins R, Wang L. Contribution of posterior corneal astigmatism. J Cataract Refract Surg. 2012;38(12):2080–7.
2. Felipe A, Artigas JM, Díez-Ajenjo A, García-Domene C, Alcocer P. Residual astigmatism produced by toric intraocular lens rotation. J Cataract Refract Surg. 2011;37(10):1895–901.

Apps and Social Networking Pages for Glaucoma

4

Glaucoma being a disease that requires lifelong medical management and strict compliance is one of the best candidates for app development. Mobile devices have been used for intraocular pressure (IOP) assessment and recording to screening of disc photographs [1]. With the sudden boom in mobile augmented imaging of the optic disc for screening of patients to rapid assessment of visual field, applications of mobile computing to diagnosis and management of glaucoma are bound to increase with time [2, 3]. We shall review the best available current applications on Android and iOS platforms that can be easily adapted into the daily workflow of your glaucoma practice.

Applications

The App pages can broadly be divided into four categories:

A. Patient information, awareness and compliance
B. Visual field assessment
C. Physician reference and research

A. **Patient Information, Awareness and Compliance Apps**
    1. ***Glaucoma***
        - ***Platforms***: iOS and Android
        - ***App Creator***: Johannes Vegt, signs for communication
        - ***Version***: 1.3
        - ***App Size***: 5.3 MB

P. Ichhpujani, S. Thakur, *Smart Resources in Ophthalmology*, Current Practices in Ophthalmology, https://doi.org/10.1007/978-981-13-0140-7_4

- ***App Icon***:

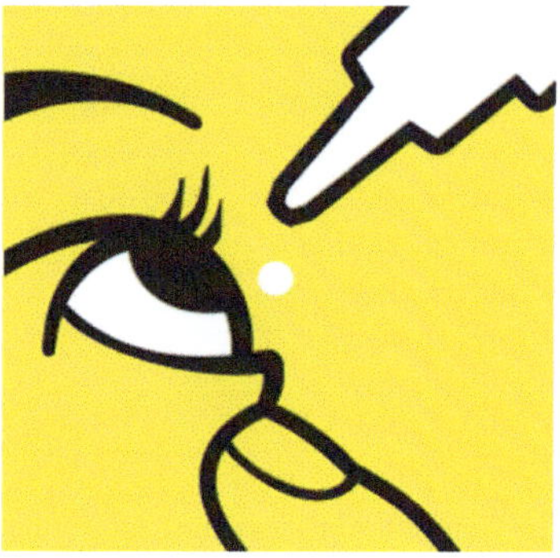

- ***App Screenshots***:

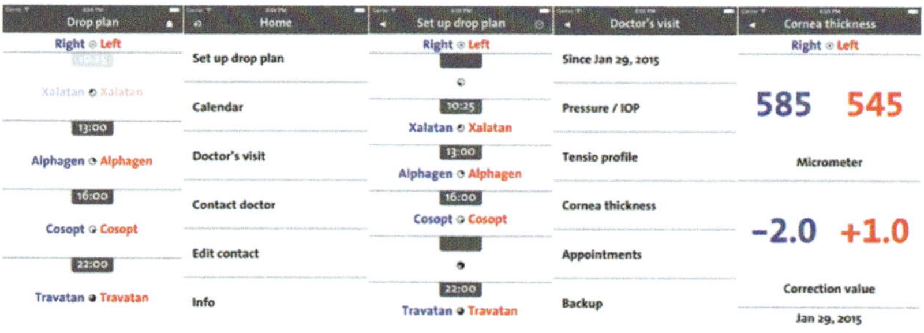

- ***Features***:
  This application provides a platform to increase the compliance of the patient. It offers tools to set up the drug regime, offers drug reminders and now even allows the patient to maintain an IOP tension profile. The application can additionally keep reminders for clinic visits. The data can be backed up in the cloud or via email. Since the application is available on both Android and iOS, it increases the flexibility and ease of usage.

  QR Scanning Codes for the App

  Android iOS

2. ***Glaucoma from Wills Eye***
   - ***Platforms***: iOS
   - ***App Creator***: Wills Eye Hospital
   - ***Version***: 1.0
   - ***App Size***: 103.5 MB
   - ***App Icon***:

Wills Eye Hospital

   - ***App Screenshots***:

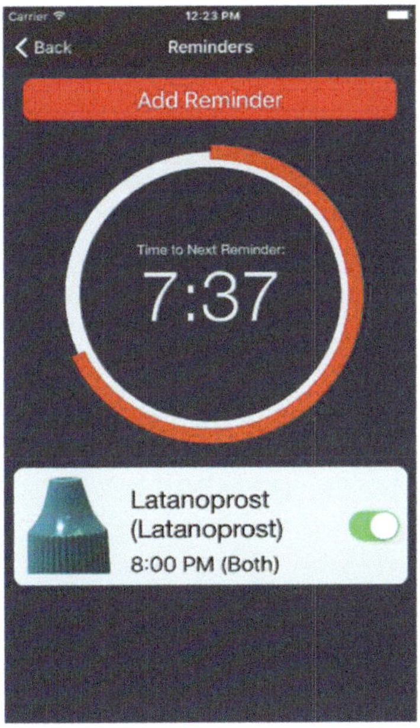

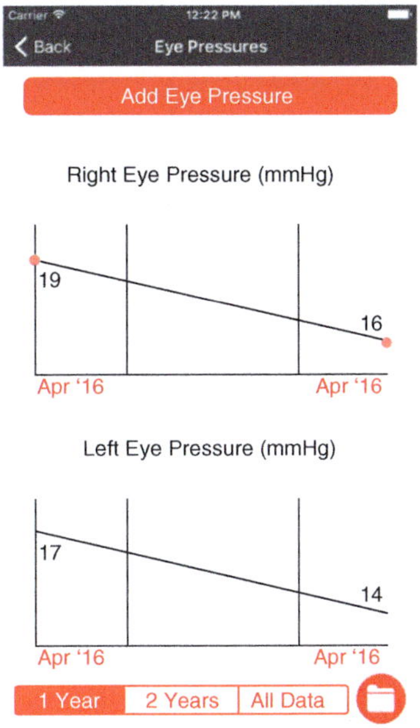

   - ***Features***:
     This application offers the best clinical advice from the glaucoma specialists at Wills Eye Hospital, Philadelphia, USA. It offers comprehensive patient information about the disease and the management options available including lasers and surgery. It also offers tools to set up the drug regime, offers drug reminders and allows the patient to maintain an IOP tension profile. The application can additionally keep reminders for clinic visits and even offers tutorials on how to effectively take a visual field exam.

QR Scanning Code for the App

3. ***Glaucoma in Perspective***
   - ***Platforms***: iOS iPad only
   - ***App Creator***: Allergan
   - ***Version***: 1.0
   - ***App Size***: 49.3 MB
   - ***App Icon***:

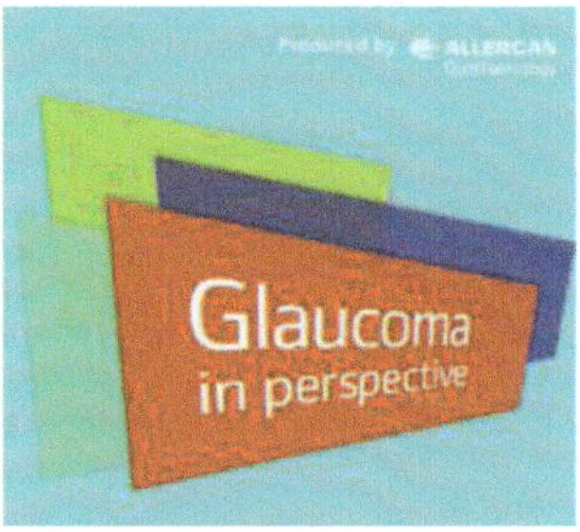

   - ***App Screenshots***:

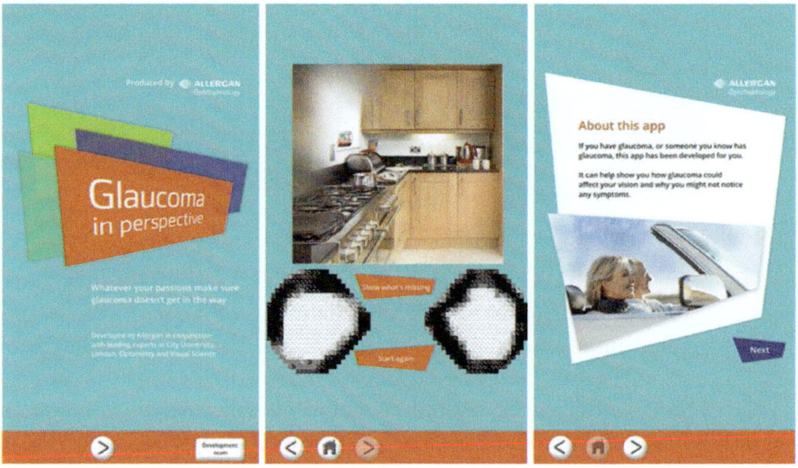

- ***Features***:
  This application provides patient information about glaucoma in an attractive package. From visual field contraction tool to information about anti-glaucoma drugs and glaucoma risk factors, this application is an easy alternative to lengthy discussions at the clinic about the disease and what to expect during treatment and follow-up.

  QR Scanning Code for the App

B. **Visual Field Assessment**
   1. ***Visual Fields Easy***
      - ***Platforms***: iOS (iPad only)
      - ***App Creator***: George Kong Softwares
      - ***Version***: 8.1
      - ***App Size***: 16.1 MB
      - ***App Icon***:

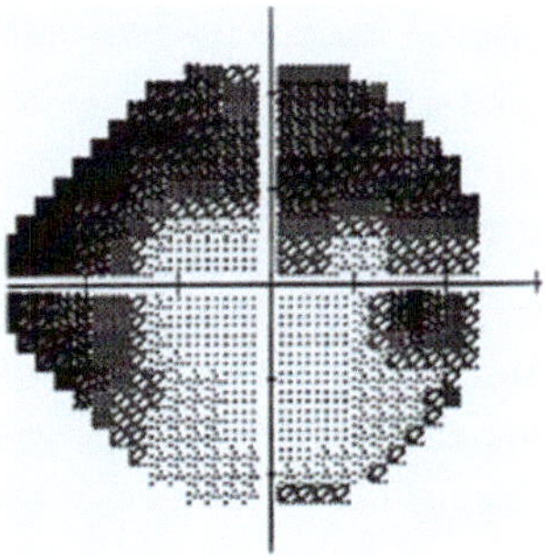

- ***App Screenshot***:

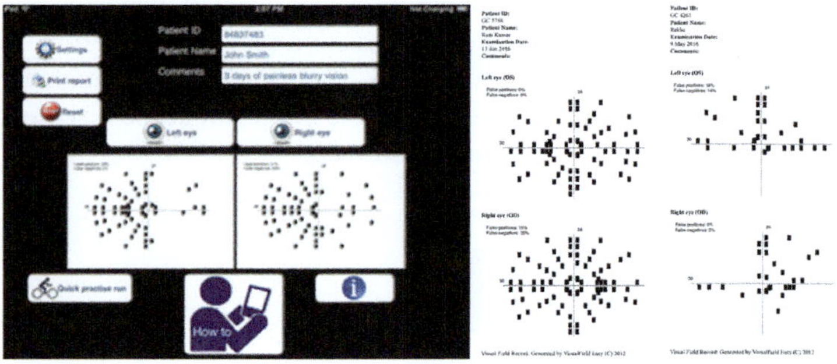

- ***Features***:
  This application uses the suprathreshold method of visual fields testing to detect gross abnormalities in the visual fields. The results have to be analysed using a coder software that provides missed points and false positives/negatives. The application offers a simple and fast way for visual field assessment but has been superseded by MRF application that provides better data for comparative assessment with the conventional Humphrey visual fields. The screenshots above show the VFE output for patients of moderate and severe glaucoma. Recently published results show that the Visual Fields Easy test procedure is a portable, fast, effective procedure for detecting moderate and advanced visual field loss [4]. The application also has been demonstrated to be useful in monitoring field loss after stroke [5].

  QR Scanning Code for the App

2. ***MRF Suite*** *(Free to $19.99)*
   - ***Platforms***: iOS (iPad only)
   - ***App Creator***: Glance Optical Pty Ltd
   - ***Version***: 2.10
   - ***App Size***: 22.3 MB
   - ***App Icon***:

- *App Screenshot*:

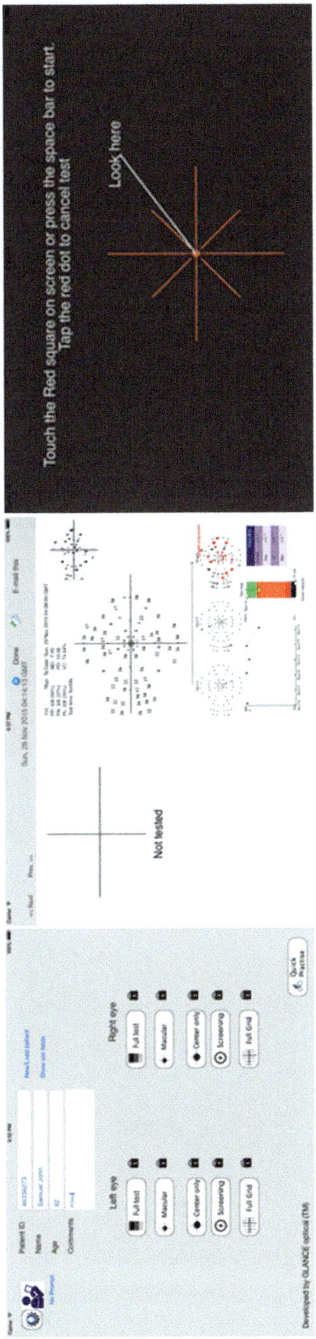

- ***Features***:
  This application offers a comprehensive assessment of visual fields. It can be used in eye conditions such as glaucoma, retinal disease and other optic neuropathies, as well as in neurological conditions (stroke, MS). MRF glaucoma has been designed to detect abnormalities in the visual field both centrally and in the periphery (up to 30° from central fixation point). Longitudinal comparison of test results is performed at the end of each test. Test results are stored and can be accessed through an online portal. Test results can be exported as comma-separated values (.CVS) format and imported into Excel for detailed point-to-point analysis (for vision research purpose). The free version allows storage for up to eight patients, and the paid version offers unlimited usage.
  MRF has been clinically validated and gives promising results in a wide range of conditions that have field loss [3, 6, 7].

  QR Scanning Code for the App

C. **Physician Reference and Research**
   1. ***Glaucoma Today***
      - ***Platforms***: iOS (iPad Only)
      - ***App Creator***: Bryn Mawr Communications LLC
      - ***Version***: 8.2
      - ***App Size***: 27.8 MB
      - ***App Icon***:

- ***App Screenshot***:

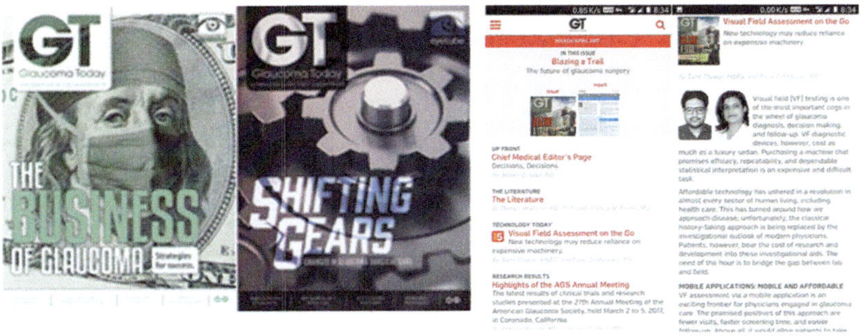

- ***Features***:
  This application offers a slick way to stay updated with everything new in the areas like recent research, surgical techniques, clinical strategies, therapeutics and technology related to glaucoma. Glaucoma Today is a bimonthly publication that profiles leaders in the field of glaucoma, and contributing authors also present challenging cases as a source of education for readers. It is also available online in a mobile-optimized format via http://glaucomatoday.com.

  QR Scanning Code for the App

2. ***Glaucoma Calc ($1.99)***
   - ***Platforms***: iOS (iOS and iWatch compatible)
   - ***App Creator***: Optical Directions Consulting
   - ***Version***: 1.7
   - ***App Size***: 8.7 MB
   - ***App Icon***:

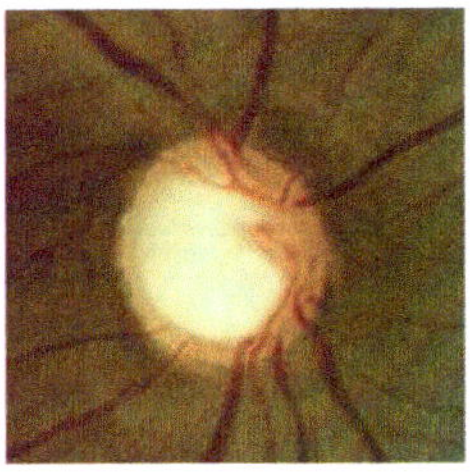

- ***App Screenshots***:

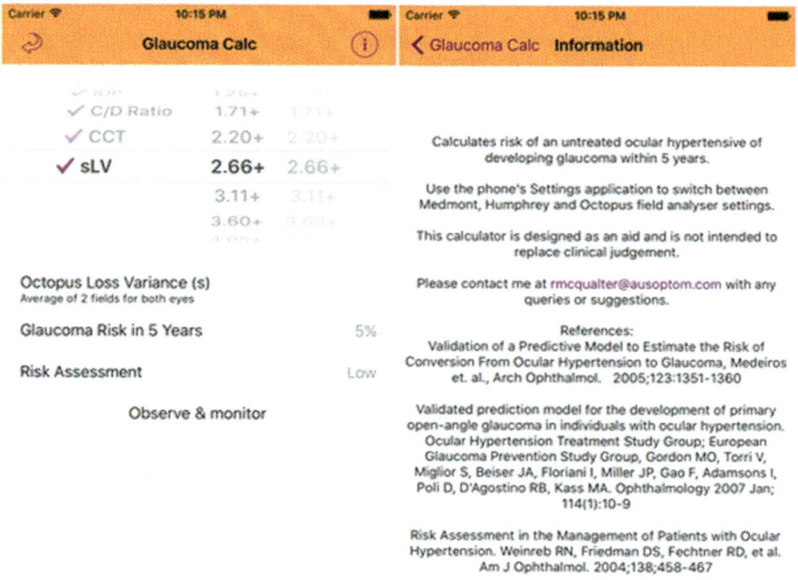

- ***Features***:
  This application offers full support for all three major perimeters: Humphrey, Medmont and Octopus. Simple to use, it uses five parameters (Age, IOP, C/D ratio, CCT and PSD/PD/LV) to display the glaucoma risk. The calculator is based on the OHTS (Ocular Hypertension Treatment Study) and has been clinically validated [8].

  QR Scanning Code for the App

3. ***Glaucoma Pro***
   - ***Platforms***: Android
   - ***App Creator***: Chad Cozart
   - ***Version***: 1.7
   - ***App Size***: 8.7 MB

- ***App Icon***:

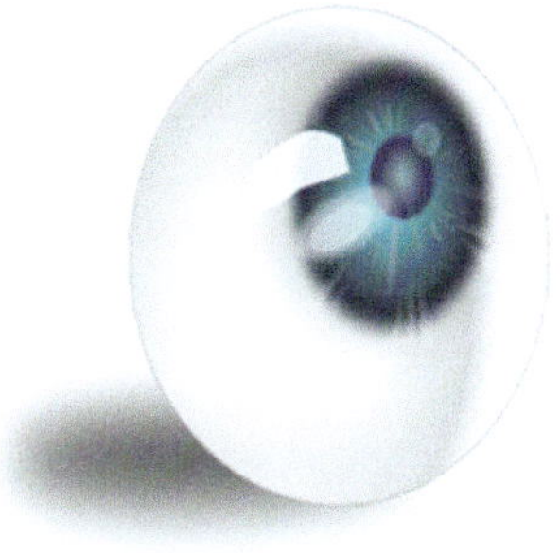

- ***App Screenshots***:

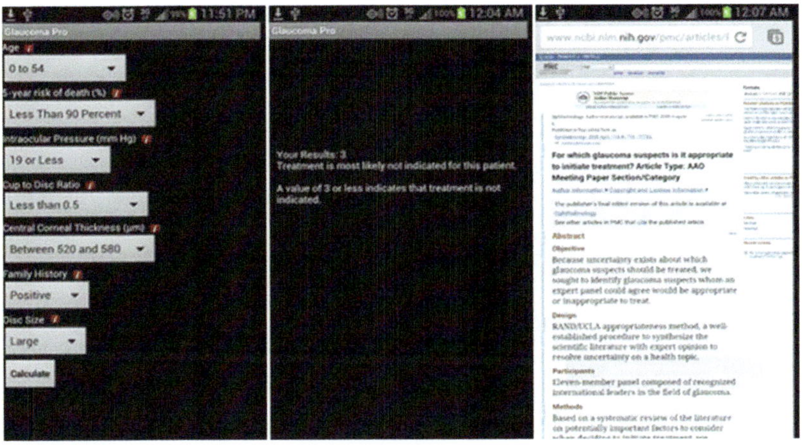

- ***Features***:
  This application uses seven parameters (age, life expectancy, intraocular pressure (IOP), central corneal thickness, cup-disc ratio, disc size and family history) to calculate the need for initiation of treatment in a glaucoma patient. The calculator is based on Appropriateness of Treating Glaucoma Suspects RAND Study Group [9].

  QR Scanning Code for the App

4. ***Glaucoma*** *(Free with In-App Purchase)*
   - ***Platforms***: Android
   - ***App Creator***: Focus Medica
   - ***Version***: 2.3
   - ***App Size***: 17.75 MB
   - ***App Icon***:

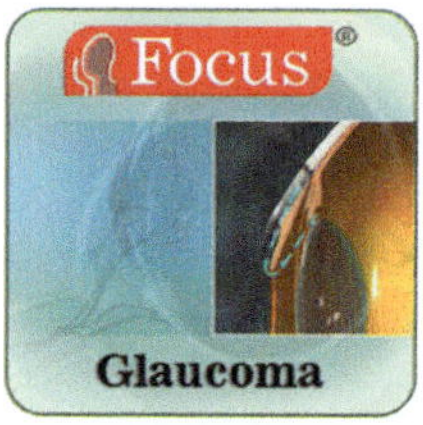

   - ***App Screenshot***:

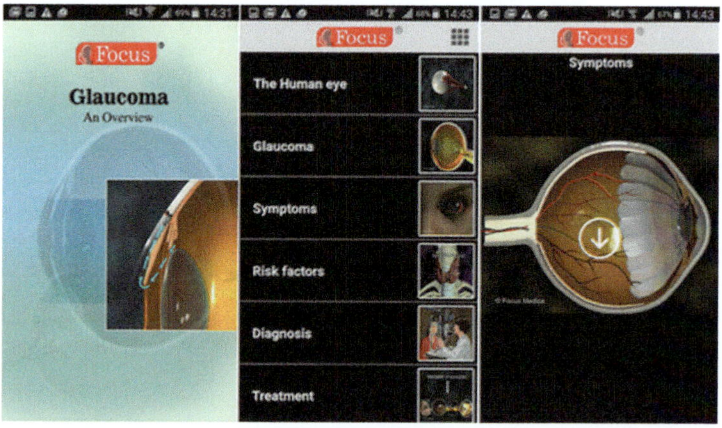

   - ***Features***:
     This application helps in understanding the disease condition through animated videos. Different animations in the application describe the anatomy of the eye, particularly related to draining of the aqueous humour, and the various causes that lead to glaucoma, highlighting the diagnostic and treatment options available.

     QR Scanning Code for the App

5. ***Spectralis***
   - ***Platforms***: iOS
   - ***App Creator***: Heidelberg Engineering GmbH
   - ***Version***: 4.0
   - ***App Size***: 52.2 MB
   - ***App Icon***:

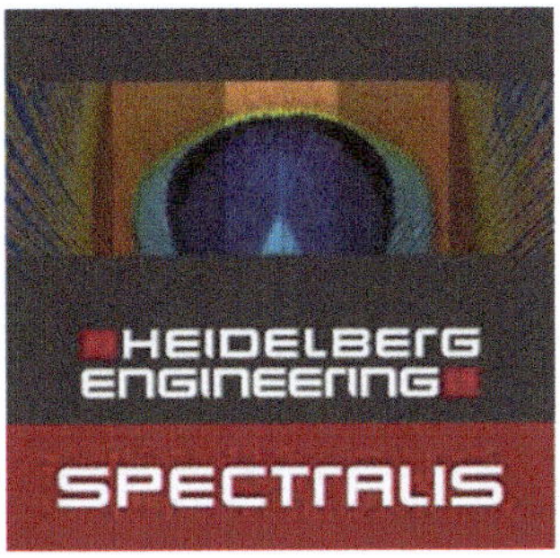

   - ***App Screenshot***:

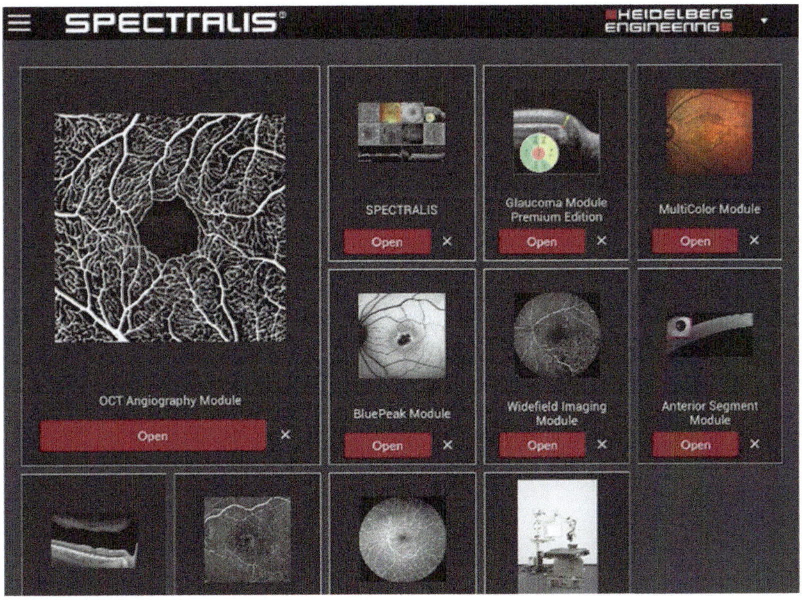

   - ***Features***:
     The official Spectralis application provides easy access to a broad range of comprehensive information about the retina and glaucoma-imaging platform from Heidelberg Engineering. With easy-to-understand videos, image slide shows and demonstrative medical examples, this application transcends the boundaries between disease descriptions and imaging-based diagnosis.

QR Scanning Code for the App

6. ***Target Intraocular Pressure Calculator*** *($4.99)*
    - ***Platforms***: iOS
    - ***App Creator***: Slawomir Janiec
    - ***Version***: 1.0.2
    - ***App Size***: 11.1 MB
    - ***App Icon***:

    - ***App Screenshot***:

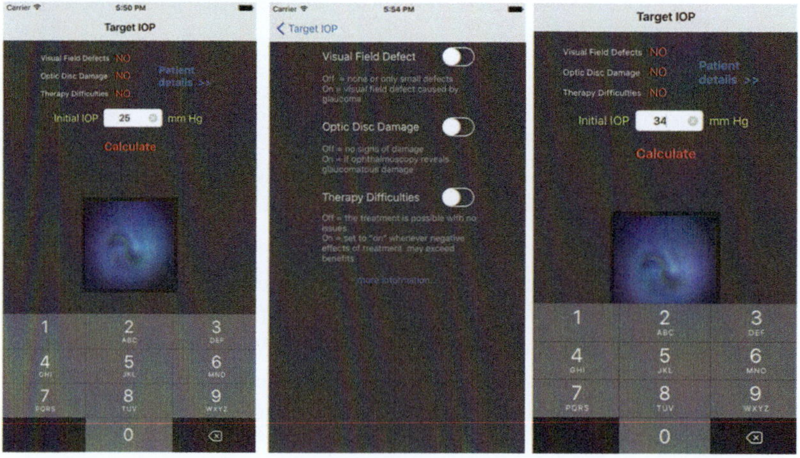

- ***Features***:

  The application provides a portable possibility to calculate the 'target intraocular pressure' in glaucoma patients. The user fills the value of initial (pretreatment) pressure and (if needed) also some basic facts describing most important patient's details. This allows to calculate the value of pressure which may be set as a target for pressure-lowering medication/treatment. The calculations are based on the target IOP calculations by Jampel [10].

  QR Scanning Code for the App

Social Networking

A. ***Web Resources***

1. ***GONE Project***: The purpose of the GONE website is to help the user understand any deficiencies in the glaucoma specialist's skills of optic nerve examination and aims to improve them with practice. The Glaucomatous Optic Neuropathy Examination (GONE) Project was developed at the Centre for Eye Research Australia and Royal Victorian Eye and Ear Hospital in Melbourne, Australia. Since 2008 GONE is on the web and is free to all, who wished to test themselves on their examination skills of the optic nerve head. The results have been published, and they concluded that ophthalmology trainees and comprehensive ophthalmologists underestimated glaucoma likelihood in approximately one in five disc photographs and were twice as likely to underestimate as overestimate glaucoma likelihood. Underestimating the vertical cup-disc ratio and cup shape and missing retinal nerve fibre layer defects and disc haemorrhage were the key errors that led to underestimation [11]. A partner application has also been developed for the iPad, which allows the GONE project to be used in an applet form.

Website Screenshots

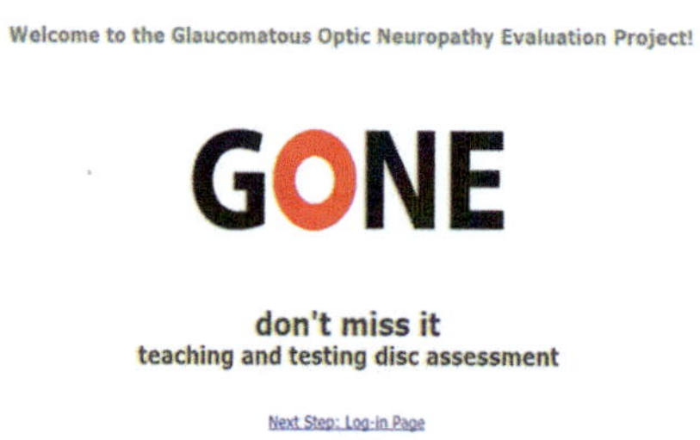

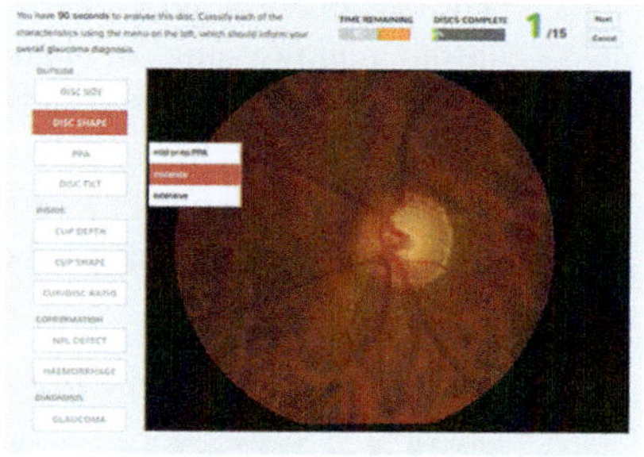

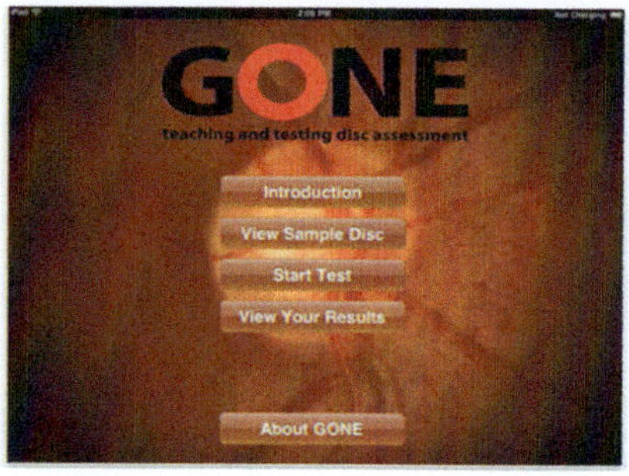

Site URL: http://www.gone-project.com

2. ***World Glaucoma Association (WGA) and its associate websites***: In addition to organizing the annual World Glaucoma Congress, the WGA also comes out with the International Glaucoma Review (IGR). It is a 3-monthly publication of a critical review—the Editors Selection—and classified abstracts of all glaucoma literature, in addition, reports, meeting announcements, comments and views. If its glaucoma, IGR has it. The activities of WGA help in increasing the availability and knowledge of glaucoma literature. It also increases the cooperation and reporting of WGA-affiliated glaucoma societies and has become the one-stop solution to gather knowledge about current research in glaucoma. The WGA also organizes the widely popular World Glaucoma Week (March 11–17 annually), and its website provides easy-to-assimilate information for patients and physicians alike.

Website Screenshots

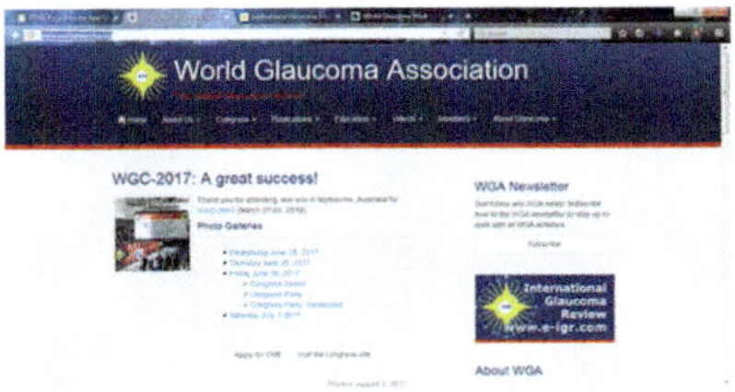

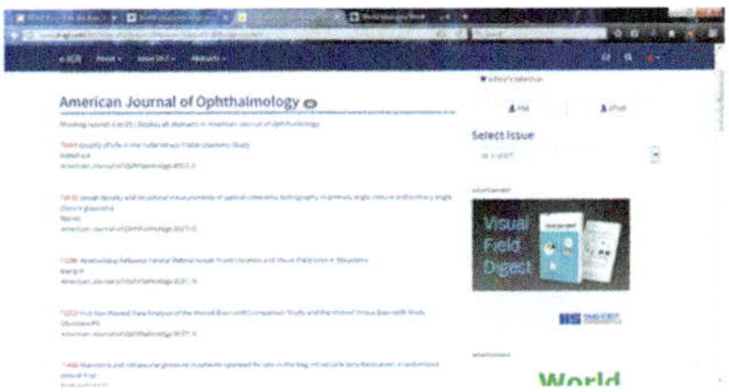

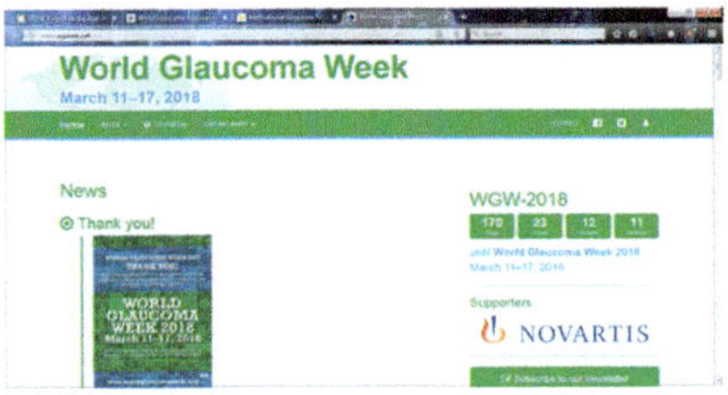

Site URL: **http*://www.worldglaucoma.org, http://www.wgweek.net and http://www.e-igr.com***

3. ***Glaucoma Australia***: One of the best Internet resources for patient information about glaucoma. Their information is well sorted out and is even available as free downloadable PDFs in 13 languages.

   Website Screenshots

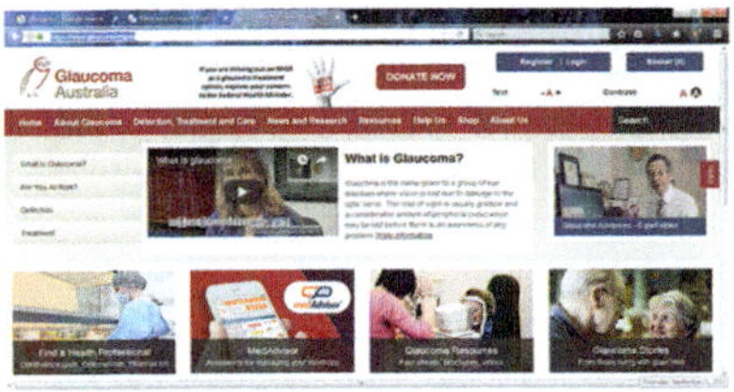

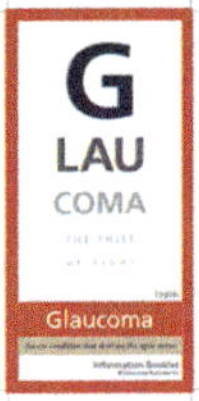

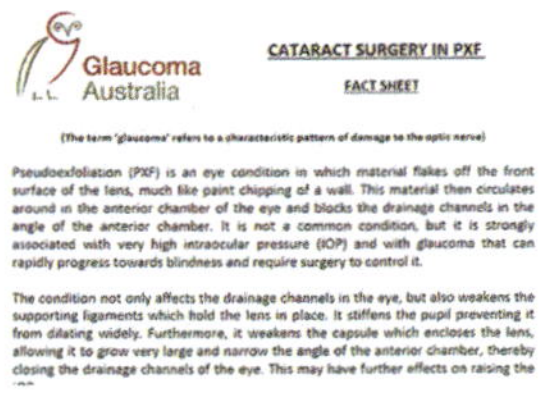

Site URL: https://www.glaucoma.org.au

B. ***Facebook Pages***

S. No	Page icon	Page name	Description	QR code
Glaucoma society pages				
1.		ISGS: International Society of Glaucoma Surgery	The International Society of Glaucoma Surgery is a non-governmental, non-profit organization that aims at promoting the art and science of glaucoma surgery, through active dissemination of knowledge and support of education and research	
2.		European Glaucoma Society	Founded in 1978, EGS is at the forefront of glaucoma research and education. This page keeps you updated with EGS events, tip of the months and current high-impact articles	
3.		American Glaucoma Society	Founded in 1985, AGS promotes excellence in the care of patients with glaucoma and preserves or enhances vision by supporting glaucoma specialists and scientists through the advancement of education and research	
4.	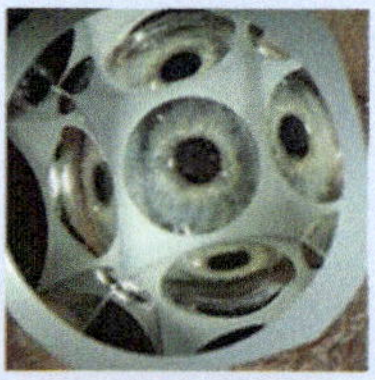	Glaucoma International Forum	Fostering international exchange of ideas and networking for eye care providers, this is the official AAO forum	
5.		World Glaucoma Association	Since 2002, WGA is an independent, impartial, ethical, global organization for glaucoma science and care	

S. No	Page icon	Page name	Description	QR code
Journal pages				
1.	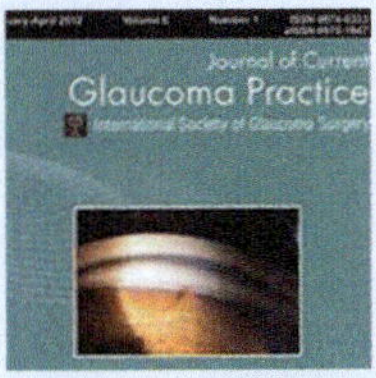	Journal of Current Glaucoma Practice	Official page of the Journal of Current Glaucoma Practice	
2.		National Journal of Glaucoma	Official page of the Russian Journal of Glaucoma	
3.		Glaucoma Today	Official page of Glaucoma Today	
Physician information and training				
1.		Glaucoma Guru	Brainchild of Dr Tarek Shaarawy, this page has loads of surgical techniques, diagnostic pearls and high-quality clinical vignettes from one of the most respected names in glaucoma research and treatment	
Patient support groups				
1.		Glaucoma Australia	Founded in 1988, Glaucoma Australia is a national, not-for-profit registered charity dedicated to raising awareness about glaucoma and to support glaucoma sufferers	

(continued)

S. No	Page icon	Page name	Description	QR code
2.		International Glaucoma Association	Founded in 1974, the IGA is a charity for people with glaucoma. They provide information, literature and advice and fund essential research to prevent unnecessary loss of sight through early detection, diagnosis and treatment	
3.		Support Glaucoma Research	Created by a glaucoma patient, Sonal Sathe, this page is regularly updated with glaucoma awareness articles	
4.		World Glaucoma Week	March 12–18 every year is celebrated as the World Glaucoma Week; this page updates activity done across the world for glaucoma awareness	
5.		World Glaucoma Patient Association	The official page of the World Glaucoma Patient Association	

C. *Twitter Handles*

S. No	Handle icon	Handle name	Description	QR code
1.	GLAUCOMA	Glaucoma	Handle provides glaucoma information, screening, detection glaucoma events, news and clinical updates	
2.	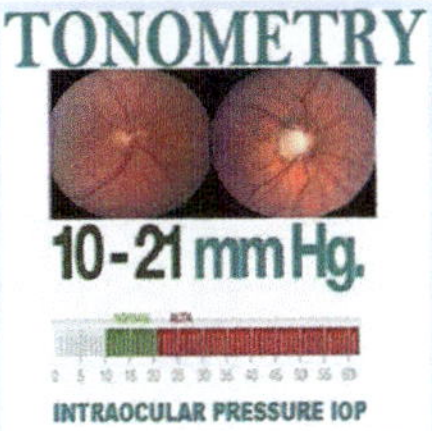	Tonometry	Gives information about IOP, glaucoma, blindness and glaucoma awareness	
3.	IGR	International Glaucoma Review	International Glaucoma Review—The Journal of the World Glaucoma Association	
4.	GT Glaucoma Today	Glaucoma Today	Glaucoma Today delivers important information on recent research, surgical techniques, clinical strategies, therapeutics and technology	
5.	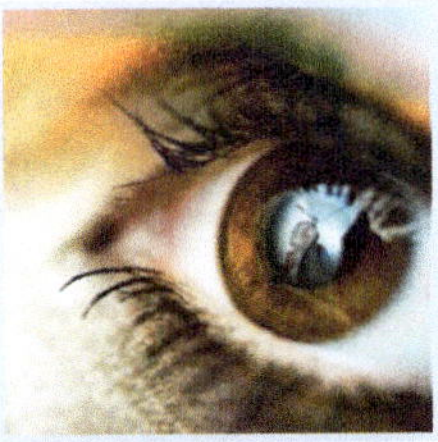	Glaucoma Foundation	The Glaucoma Foundation's mission is to develop a cure for glaucoma through innovative research and collaboration	
6.	G	Glaucoma Research Foundation	Glaucoma Research Foundation is a non-profit dedicated to funding innovative research, and providing education and support	

(continued)

S. No	Handle icon	Handle name	Description	QR code
7.		American Glaucoma Society	Founded in 1985, AGS promotes excellence in the care of patients with glaucoma and preserves or enhances vision by supporting glaucoma specialists and scientists through the advancement of education and research	
8.		World Glaucoma Association	Since 2002, WGA is an independent, impartial, ethical, global organization for glaucoma science and care	
9.		International Glaucoma Association	Founded in 1974, the IGA is a charity for people with glaucoma. They provide information, literature and advice and fund essential research to prevent unnecessary loss of sight through early detection, diagnosis and treatment	
10.		World Glaucoma Week	March 12–18 every year is celebrated as the World Glaucoma Week; this page updates activity done across the world for glaucoma awareness	
11.		Asia Pacific Glaucoma Society	The official twitter handle of the Asia Pacific Glaucoma Society	

S. No	Handle icon	Handle name	Description	QR code
12.		Childhood Glaucoma Network	Childhood Glaucoma Network is where all people affected by childhood glaucoma come to share their story	

Mobile Perimetry

Mobile applications that allow visual field charting have opened up an exciting avenue in glaucoma research. There are several other powerful tools that are available for visual field charting on laptops and desktops. With the increasing use of 3D and virtual reality in developing novel perimeters, it is imperative that glaucoma diagnosis indeed has a bright future [12–14]. Some of these programmes are described below:

1. **SPARCS**: The Spaeth/Richman contrast sensitivity test is a new way to measure contrast sensitivity. Its efficacy and reliability have been demonstrated in comparison to the conventional Pelli-Robson chart test [15]. What makes SPARCS different is the ability to test peripheral contrast sensitivity that gives us an estimate of glaucomatous damage [16]. This has also been demonstrated in published literature. In addition to glaucoma, SPARCS has also been used to test contrast sensitivity in patients of cataract, ARMD and refractive error [17–19].

   Website Screenshots

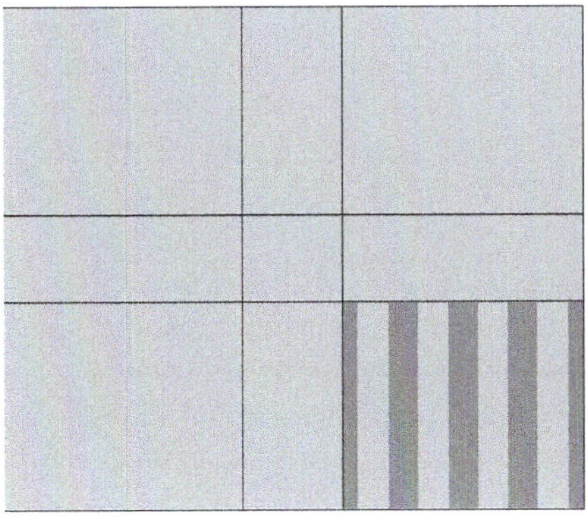

Testing Screen

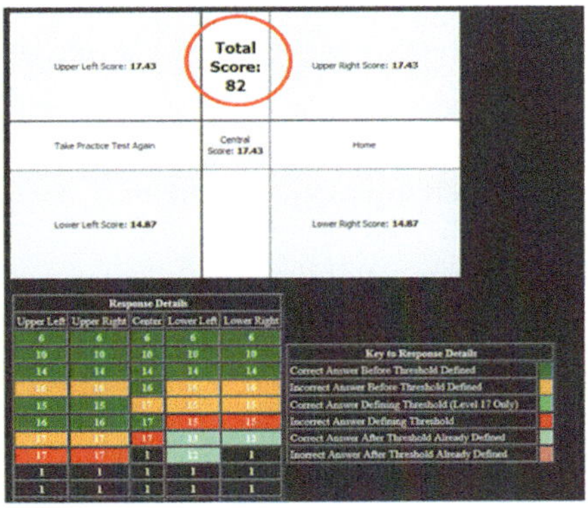

Result Screen

   Site URL: https://www.sparcscontrastcenter.com/home.php

2. **Peristat**: Peristat is an achromatic static computer threshold testing programme. It has been compared to the Humphrey visual field (HVF) 24-2 SITA standard testing and has showed good results [20]. The test is available online and can be taken at the office or at home. Peristat has been shown to have a sensitivity ranging from 80 to 83% [21]. Self-administered home-based Peristat has been shown to have comparable efficacy in detecting scotomas as office-based testing under clinical supervision and thus has the potential to be used as a self-administered home screening perimetric test [22].

   Website Screenshots

   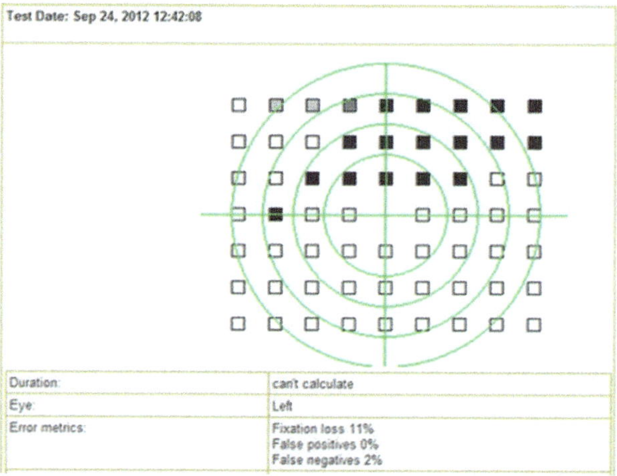

   ***Site URL**: http://www.keepyoursight.org/peristat.php*

3. **VR or Head Held Perimeters**: Binocular testing using head held perimeters has also been tried for visual field assessment with success. Prototypes include the Kasha visual field system, the Virtual Eye system and the latest Android-based VR-assisted visual field application [14, 23, 24]. The results of these mobile perimeters have been very promising, and they may soon replace the conventional Humphrey visual fields.

With the advent of these mobile perimeters, teleglaucoma will become a more viable alternative for diagnosis and treatment of glaucomas in resource-poor countries. A recent meta-analysis has pointed out that teleglaucoma (the use of stereoscopic digital imaging to take ocular images, which are transmitted electronically to an ocular specialist) is more specific but less sensitive than in-person examination. The pooled estimate of sensitivity was 0.832 [95% CI 0.770, 0.881], and specificity was 0.790 [95% CI 0.668, 0.876]. Teleglaucoma has also been shown to reduce patient travel times by 61 h and physician wait times by 30% in comparison to in-person examination. Additionally teleglaucoma is more cost-effective than in-person examination with an ICER (incremental cost-effectiveness ratio) of $27,460/QALY indicating that teleglaucoma will save $27,460 for each additional QALY gained. These numbers indicate that teleglaucoma is a viable alternative to in-person examination and can be pursued as a viable avenue of teleophthalmology [2, 25]. The addition of mobile perimetry to the teleglaucoma repertoire promises that the future of glaucoma care is more easy, effective and efficient.

References

1. Moradian S, Safi S. Application of mobile phones in ophthalmology. J Ophthalmic Vis Res. 2015;10(2):200–5.
2. Thomas SM, Jeyaraman MM, Hodge WG, Hutnik C, Costella J, Malvankar-Mehta MS. The effectiveness of teleglaucoma versus in-patient examination for glaucoma screening: a systematic review and meta-analysis. PLoS One. 2014;9(12):e113779.
3. Vingrys AJ, Healey JK, Liew S, Saharinen V, Tran M, Wu W, et al. Clinical validation of a tablet perimeter. In: 2016 annual meeting of the Association for Research in Vision and Ophthalmology (ARVO), Seattle, WA, 3 May 2016.
4. Johnson CA, Thapa S, George Kong YX, Robin AL. Performance of an iPad application to detect moderate and advanced visual field loss in Nepal. Am J Ophthalmol. 2017;182:147–54.
5. Spofforth J, Codina C, Bjerre A. Is the 'visual fields easy' application a useful tool to identify visual field defects in patients who have suffered a stroke? Ophthalmol Res. 2017;7(1):1–10.
6. Kong YXG, He M, Crowston JG, Vingrys AJ. A comparison of perimetric results from a tablet perimeter and Humphrey Field Analyzer in glaucoma patients. Transl Vis Sci Technol. 2016;5(6):2.
7. Nesaratnam N, Thomas PBM, Kirollos R, Vingrys AJ, Kong GYX, Martin KR. Tablets at the bedside - iPad-based visual field test used in the diagnosis of Intrasellar Haemangiopericytoma: a case report. BMC Ophthalmol. 2017;17(1):53.
8. Medeiros FA, Weinreb RN, Sample PA, Gomi CF, Bowd C, Crowston JG, et al. Validation of a predictive model to estimate the risk of conversion from ocular hypertension to glaucoma. Arch Ophthalmol. 2005;123(10):1351–60.
9. For which glaucoma suspects is it appropriate to initiate treatment? Ophthalmology. 2009;116(4):710–7.
10. Jampel HD. Target pressure in glaucoma therapy. J Glaucoma. 1997;6(2):133–8.
11. O'Neill EC, Gurria LU, Pandav SS, Kong YX, Brennan JF, Xie J, et al. Glaucomatous optic neuropathy evaluation project: factors associated with underestimation of glaucoma likelihood. JAMA Ophthalmol. 2014;132(5):560–6.
12. Nazemi PP, Fink W, Sadun AA, Francis B, Minckler D. Early detection of glaucoma by means of a novel 3D computer-automated visual field test. Br J Ophthalmol. 2007;91(10):1331–6.
13. Nguyen DT, Fahimi A, Fink W, Nazemi PP, Kim JK, Sadun AA. Novel 3D computer-automated threshold Amsler grid visual field testing of scotomas in patients with glaucoma. Eur J Ophthalmol. 2009;19(5):776–82.
14. Tsapakis S, Papaconstantinou D, Diagourtas A, Droutsas K, Andreanos K, Moschos MM, et al. Visual field examination method using virtual reality glasses compared with the Humphrey perimeter. Clin Ophthalmol. 2017;11:1431–43.
15. George L. Spaeth. Validation and reproducibility of Spaeth/Richman contrast sensitivity test 2014 [updated 2015 January 29; cited 2015 October 10]. Available from: https://www.clinicaltrials.gov/ct2/show/study/NCT01300949.
16. Richman J, Zangalli C, Lu L, Wizov SS, Spaeth E, Spaeth GL. The Spaeth/Richman contrast sensitivity test (SPARCS): design, reproducibility and ability to identify patients with glaucoma. Br J Ophthalmol. 2015;99(1):16–20.
17. Sun Y, Erdem E, Lyu A, Zangalli C, Wizov SS, Lo D, et al. SPARCS: a novel assessment of contrast sensitivity and its validity in patients with refractive error. Invest Ophthalmol Vis Sci. 2014;55(13):2711.

18. Gupta L, Cvintal V, Delvadia R, Sun Y, Erdem E, Zangalli C, et al. SPARCS and Pelli-Robson contrast sensitivity testing in normal controls and patients with cataract. Eye. 2017;31:753–61.
19. Faria BM, Duman F, Zheng CX, Waisbourd M, Gupta L, Ali M, et al. Evaluating contrast sensitivity in age-related macular degeneration using a novel computer-based test, the Spaeth/Richman contrast sensitivity test. Retina. 2015;35(7):1465–73.
20. Lowry EA, Hou J, Hennein L, Chang RT, Lin S, Keenan J, et al. Comparison of peristat online perimetry with the Humphrey perimetry in a clinic-based setting. Transl Vis Sci Technol. 2016;5(4):4.
21. Ianchulev T, Pham P, Makarov V, Francis B, Minckler D. Peristat: a computer-based perimetry self-test for cost-effective population screening of glaucoma. Curr Eye Res. 2005;30(1):1–6.
22. Wang S, Hou J, Ianchulev S, Chon B, Han Y, Chang R. Clinical utility of web-based office and home peristat for the detection of visual field defects in patients with glaucoma. Invest Ophthalmol Vis Sci. 2013;54(15):3958.
23. Hollander D, Volpe N, Moster M, Liu G, Balcer L, Judy K, et al. Use of a portable head mounted perimetry system to assess bedside visual fields. Br J Ophthalmol. 2000;84(10):1185–90.
24. Wroblewski D, Francis BA, Sadun A, Vakili G, Chopra V. Testing of visual field with virtual reality goggles in manual and visual grasp modes. Biomed Res Int. 2014;2014:206082.
25. Thomas S, Hodge W, Malvankar-Mehta M. The cost-effectiveness analysis of teleglaucoma screening device. PLoS One. 2015;10(9):e0137913.

Apps and Social Networking Pages for Vitreoretinal and Uveal Diseases

5

Retina as a subspeciality has always been on the forefront of innovation in ophthalmology, be it new imaging techniques or simply improving modalities that are already available. This chapter gives an overview of the mobile applications that can easily improve your everyday practice. From applications that simulate view from a direct ophthalmoscope to easily useable Amsler grids, this chapter covers applications that can cater the needs of someone just starting out posterior segment examination to veterans that need that little something to take their practice to the next level.

Applications for Vitreoretina

The chapter is divided into applications that have been categorized as:

A. Physician resources
B. Resident training
C. Disease-specific applications
D. Mobile retinal imaging

A. **Physician Resources**
   1. ***Retina Today***
      - ***Platforms***: iOS and Android
      - ***App Creator***: Bryn Mawr Communications LLC
      - ***Version***: 8.2 iOS, 9.2 Android
      - ***App Size***: 27.8 MB

P. Ichhpujani, S. Thakur, *Smart Resources in Ophthalmology*, Current Practices in Ophthalmology, https://doi.org/10.1007/978-981-13-0140-7_5

- ***App Icon***:

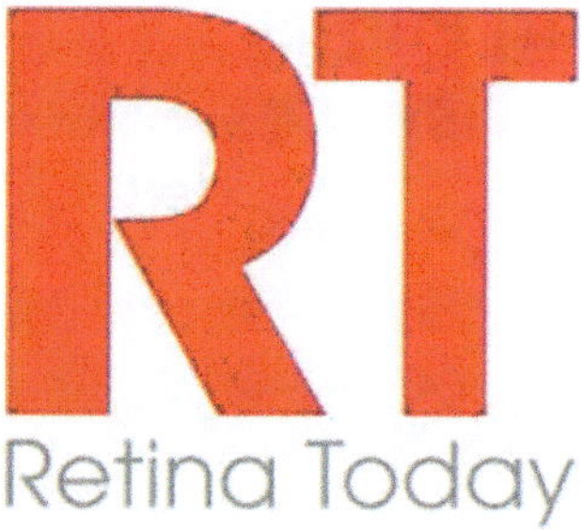

- ***App Screenshots***:

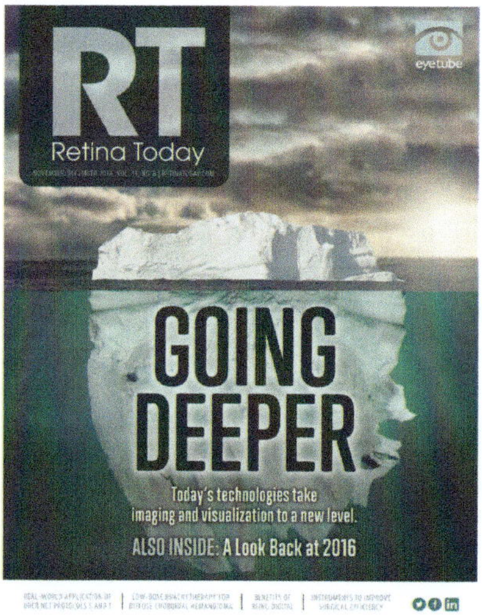

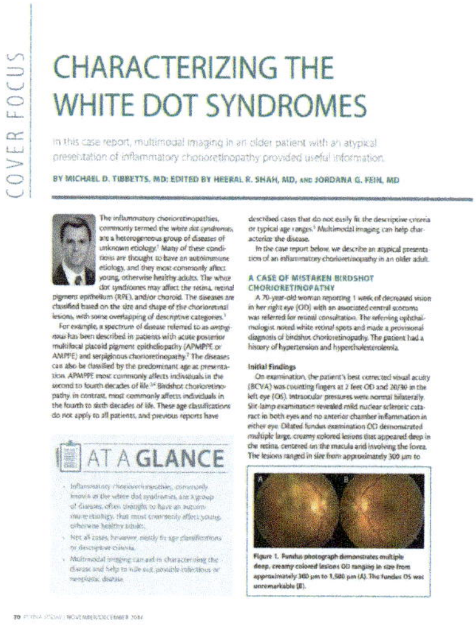

- ***Features***:

  Retina Today delivers the latest research and clinical developments addressing aspects of both the medical and surgical vitreoretina subspecialities. It also covers topics on retinal imaging, posterior segment oncology and ocular trauma. Each issue provides insight from established specialists on cutting-edge therapies and surgical techniques that are currently in use or in pipeline. The app is available both on iOS and Android and is perfect for staying updated about what's new across retina while being on the go.

QR Scanning Codes for the App

Android iOS

2. ***OSLI Retina***
   - ***Platforms***: iOS(iPhone, iPad and iPod Touch)
   - ***App Creator***: The Wyanoke Group
   - ***Version***: 1.1
   - ***App Size***: 7.4 MB
   - ***App Icon***:

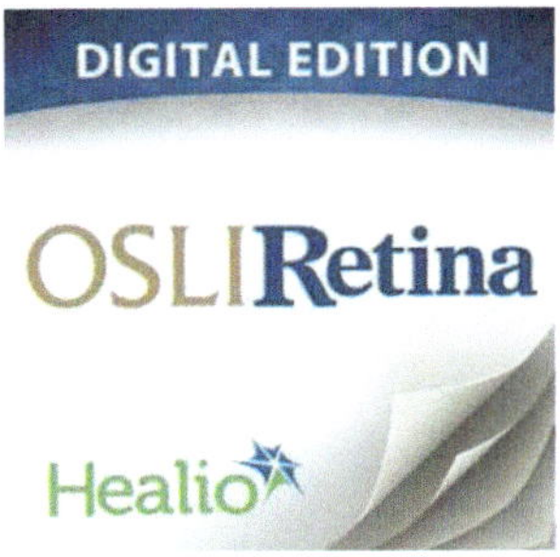

   - ***App Screenshots***:

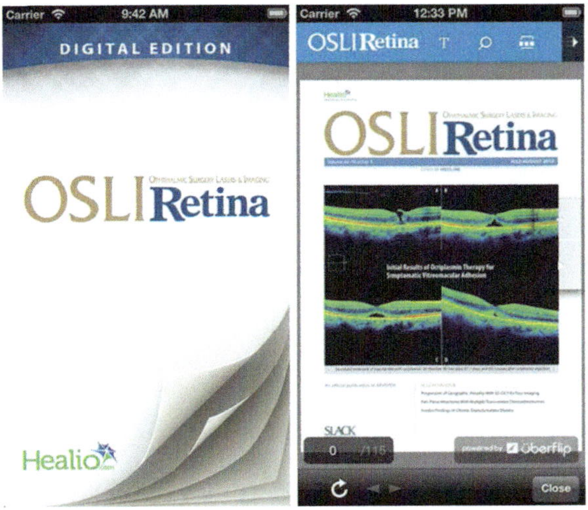

- ***Features***
  This application from the publisher of Ophthalmic Surgery Lasers and Imaging, the OSLI Retina mobile application puts the latest clinical, peer-reviewed retinal diseases, surgical and pharmacotherapy journal content at your fingertips. The application is free trial based, but continued usage requires in-application purchase of the journal subscription.
  QR Scanning Code for the App

3. ***Retina CME***
   - ***Platforms***: iOS (iPhone, iPad and iPod Touch)
   - ***App Creator***: The Wyanoke Group
   - ***Version***: 1.20
   - ***App Size***: 7.1 MB
   - ***App Icon***:

- ***App Screenshots***:

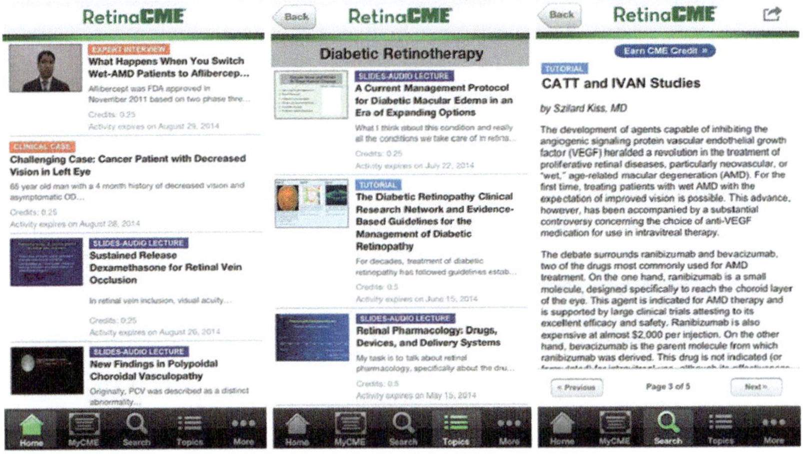

- ***Features***:
  The RetinaCME mobile app requires a free RetinaCME.com login account or registration right from the app itself. This app allows the user to earn CME credits. The user selects an activity of interest, views or listens to the study material and then completes a pre- and post-test. The CME certificate is emailed to the user once he passes the post-test. The user can also access MyCME section to see the credits he/she has earned up until that point. The activities on the RetinaCME mobile application are approved for AMA PRA Category 1 Credit(s).
  QR Scanning Code for the App

4. ***New Retina MD***
   - ***Platforms***: Android
   - ***App Creator***: Bryn Mawr Communications LLC
   - ***Version***: 8.1
   - ***App Size***: 32.95 MB

- ***App Icon***:

NRMD
New Retina MD

- ***App Screenshots***:

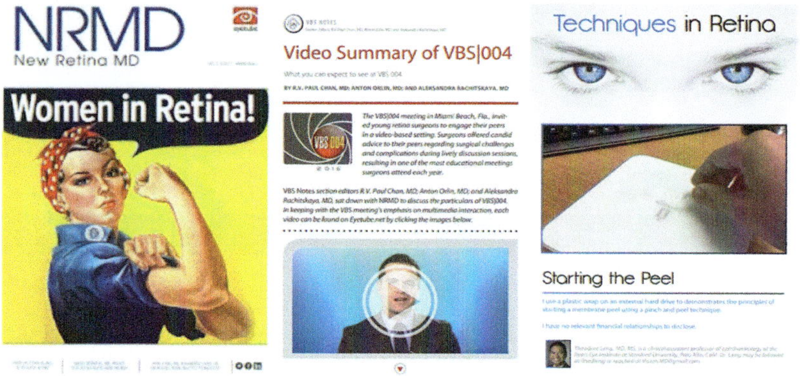

- ***Features***:
New Retina MD is a publication that delivers the latest information on clinical and non-clinical issues that are pertinent to retina specialists in their first few years of practice. This app focuses not only on surgical pearls, clinical research endeavours, practice management and continuing educational requirements but also on medical reimbursement, policy and financial planning. Each issue provides insight from the doyens in appropriate fields and is designed to fit the needs of budding physicians.
QR Scanning Code for the App

5. ***Retina World Congress***
   - ***Platforms***: iOS (iPad only)
   - ***App Creator***: CrowdCompass, Inc.
   - ***Version***: 1.1
   - ***App Size***: 73.7 MB

- ***App Icon***:

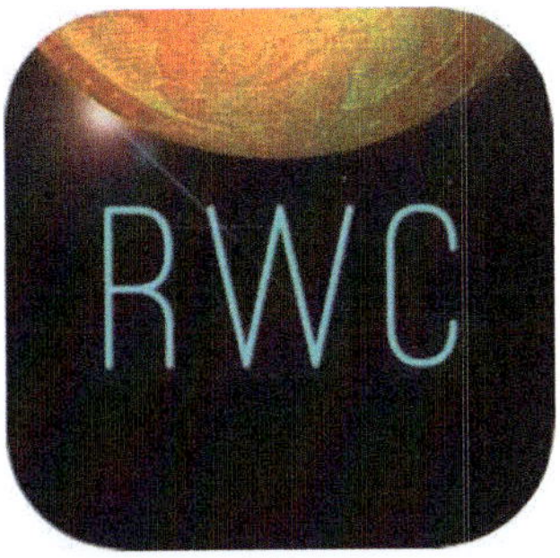

- ***App Screenshots***:

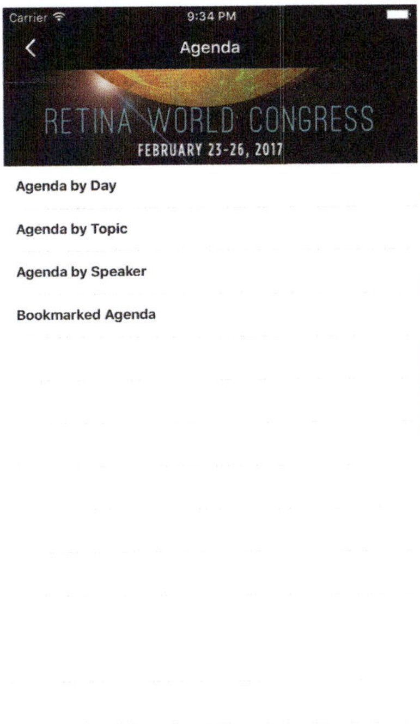

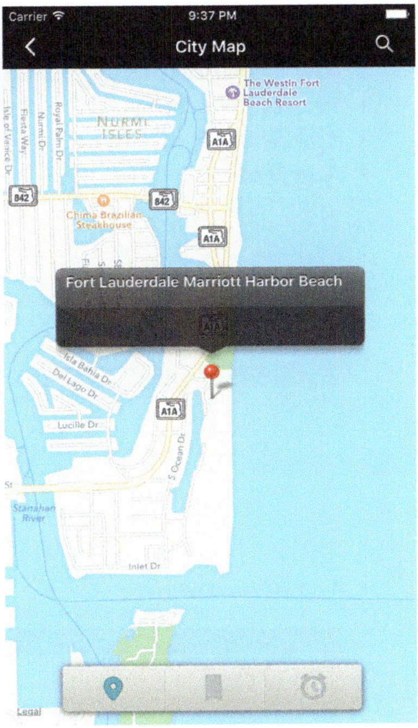

- ***Features***:
  This application is the official mobile app for Retina World Congress, one of the world's premiere educational and professional meetings for retinal specialists, which allows attendees to browse programmes and activities, create a personalized schedule and connect with colleagues.

QR Scanning Code for the App

B. **Resident Training**
   1. ***EasyScan Retina Academy***
      - ***Platforms***: iOS (iPad Only)
      - ***App Creator***: Charles Beaumont
      - ***Version***: 1.4.16
      - ***App Size***: 28 MB
      - ***App Icon***:

      - ***App Screenshots***:

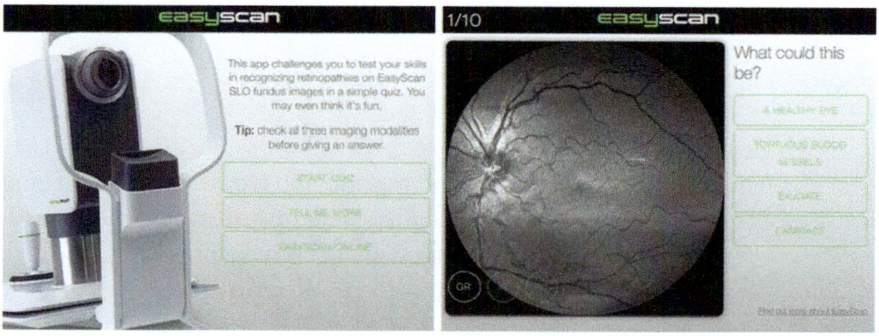

- ***Features***:
  This app challenges you to test your skills in recognizing retinopathies on EasyScan SLO fundus images in a simple quiz. The application offers a wide variety of clinical images that can help build your clinical acumen.
  QR Scanning Code for the App

2. ***Retina Base***
   - ***Platforms***: iOS and Android
   - ***App Creator***: Novartis
   - ***Version***: 1.7
   - ***App Size***: 8.7 MB
   - ***App Icon***:

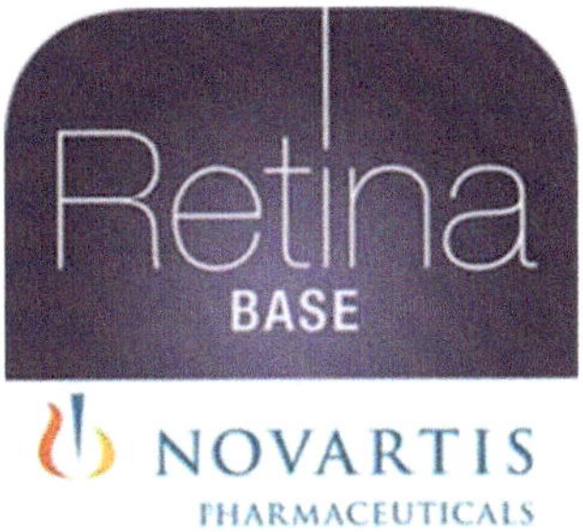

   - ***App Screenshots***:

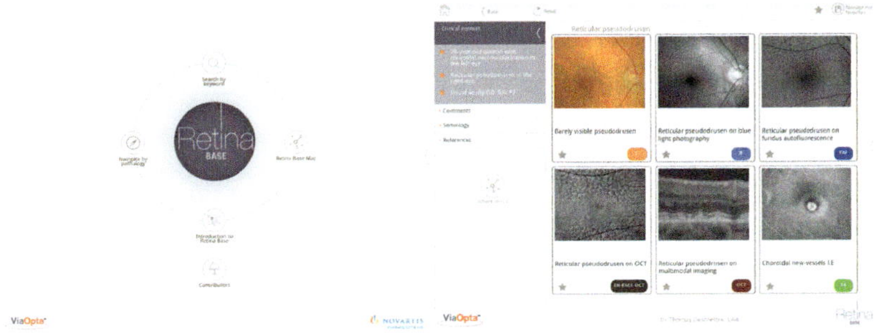

- ***Features***:
  Retina Base is a virtual library based on a myriad of clinical cases of vitreoretinal diseases. This app, developed with retina experts, allows browsing clinical cases in an intuitive way, from a typical presentation to rare versions. The application also has a keyword search engine, which may help to find the exact picture one is looking for and filter the results by category (imaging technique, pathology, clinical sign and author).
  QR Scanning Code for the App

Android iOS

3. ***Optomap UWF Retinal Imaging***
   - ***Platforms***: Android
   - ***App Creator***: Bryn Mawr Communications
   - ***Version***: 10.1
   - ***App Size***: 8.7 MB
   - ***App Icon***:

optos®

- ***App Screenshots***:

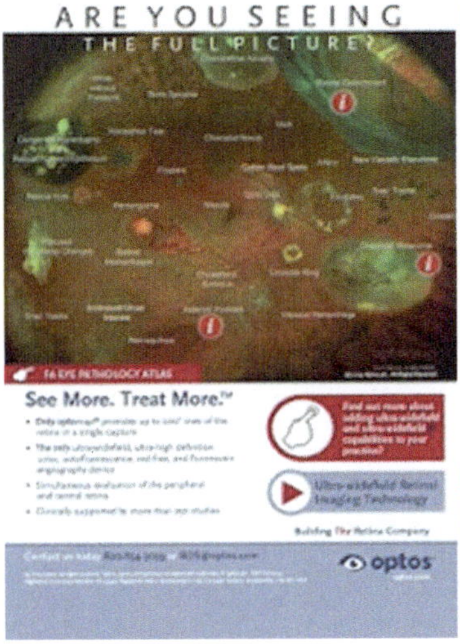

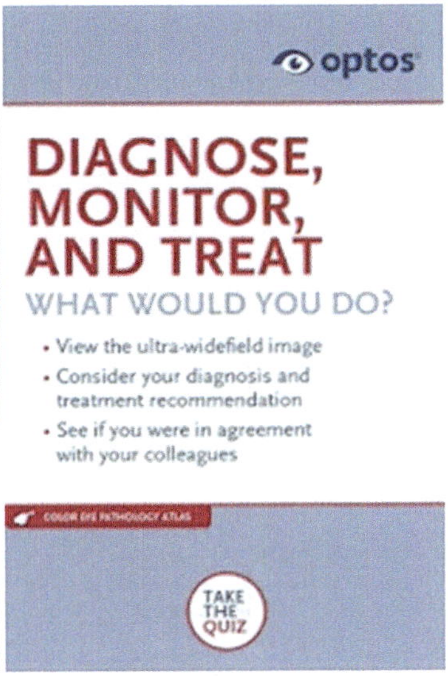

- ***Features***:
  This application sponsored by Optos is an introduction to ultrawide field imaging. With current evidence pointing out that UWF imaging is the future of retinal examination, this application makes sure you have a grasp of the abilities that this imaging modality offers [1].
  QR Scanning Code for the App

C. **Disease-Specific Applications**
   1. **Age-Related Macular Degeneration (ARMD/AMD)**
      (a) ***Eyecare Amsler Grid Eye Test***
      - ***Platforms***: iOS
      - ***App Creator***: Robert Garoon
      - ***Version***: 1.4
      - ***App Size***: 27 MB

- ***App Icon***:

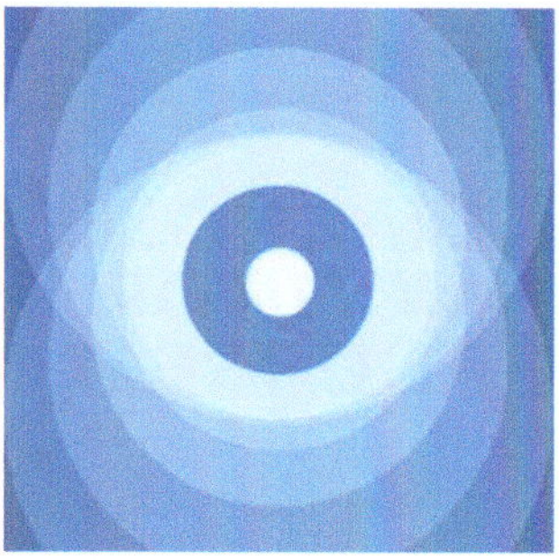

- ***App Screenshots***:

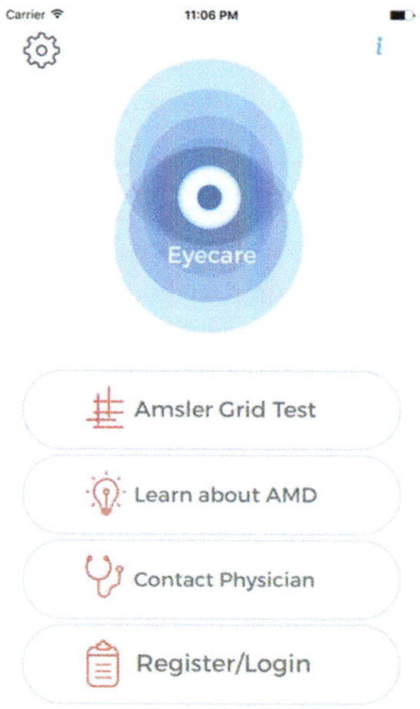

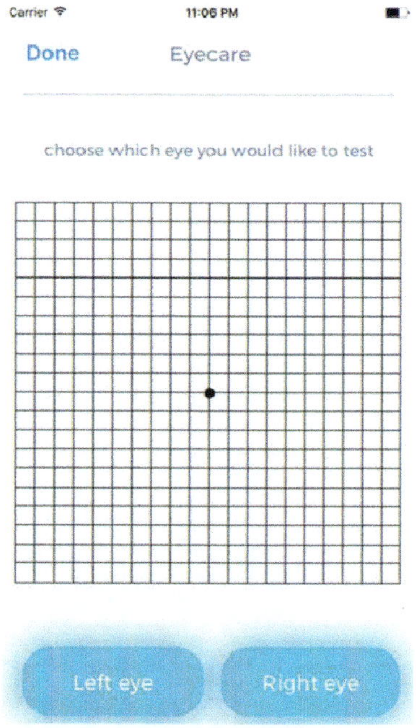

- ***Features***:
  This application is designed for personal monitoring for vision loss from macular degeneration. With daily use of the Eyecare Amsler Grid, small changes in visual function can be identified electronically that may otherwise have gone unnoticed and caused long-lasting damage. The Eyecare Amsler Grid uses proprietary technology to identify any changes in your personal Amsler grid and personally notifies you of that change almost immediately. The physicians can monitor anti-VEGF response in compliant patients, using this app.

QR Scanning Code for the App

(b) ***Amsler Grid Test***

- ***Platforms***: Android
- ***App Creator***: LVPEI-MITRA
- ***Version***: 2.1
- ***App Size***: 1.99 MB
- ***App Icon***:

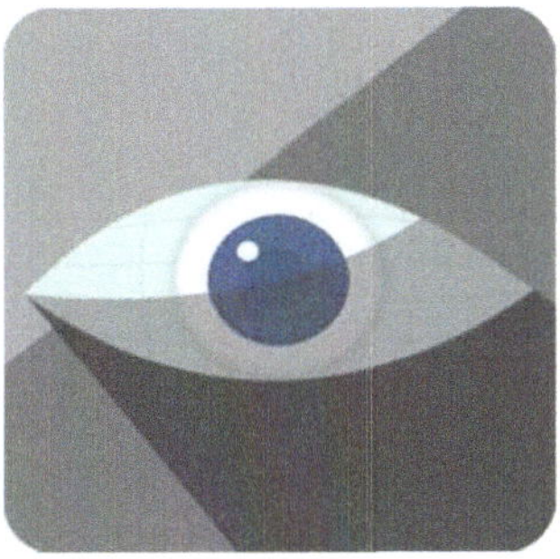

- ***App Screenshots***:

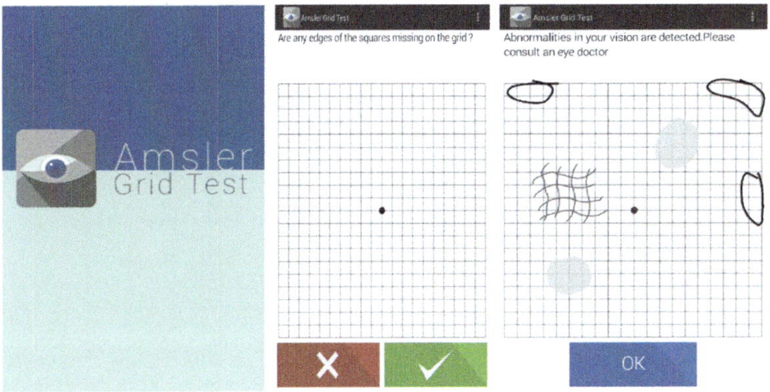

- ***Features***:
  This interactive application allows the patient to interactively draw distorted areas of the grid. Audio-guided instructions are also available. The application stores the results on the device and keeps record of them. Additionally the patient can email the patterns to the physician.
  QR Scanning Code for the App

(c) ***Amsler Grids ($9.99)***
- ***Platforms***: iOS
- ***App Creator***: Konan Medical USA
- ***Version***: 1.1
- ***App Size***: 2.6 MB
- ***App Icon***:

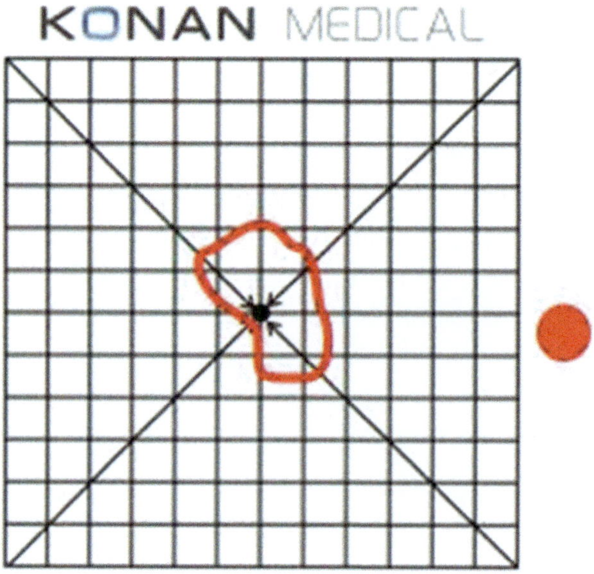

- ***App Screenshots***:

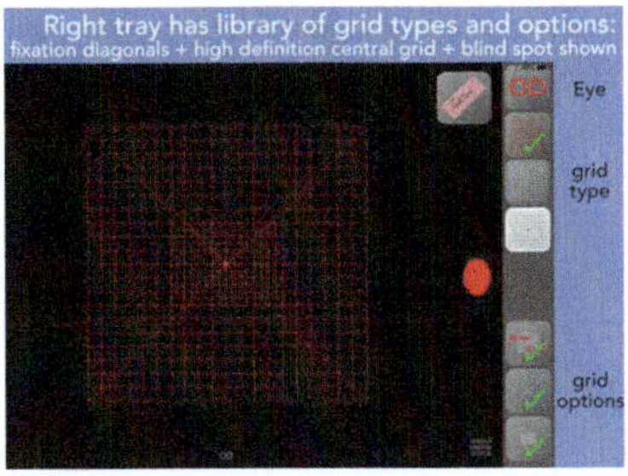

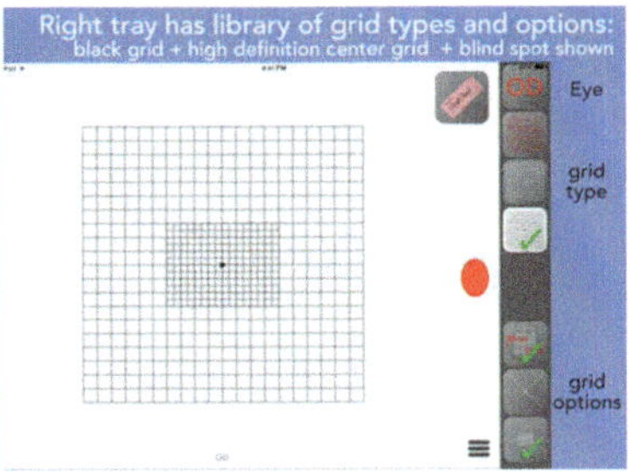

- ***Features***:
  This is a simple-to-use Amsler grid with uniquely flexible test types offering white grid on black background, red grid on black background and black grid on white background. The results can be saved for future reference within the application.
  QR Scanning Code for the App

(d) ***AMD—A Metamorphopsia Detector ($3.99iOS, free trial on Android)***

- ***Platforms***: iOS and Android
- ***App Creator***: app4eyes
- ***Version***: 1.2
- ***App Size***: 1 MB
- ***App Icon***:

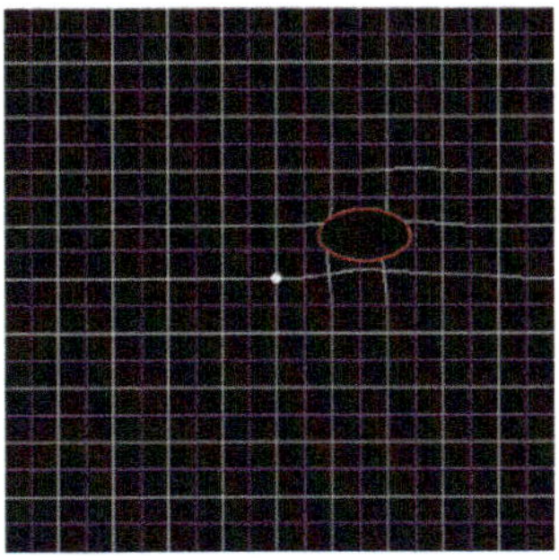

- ***App Screenshots***:

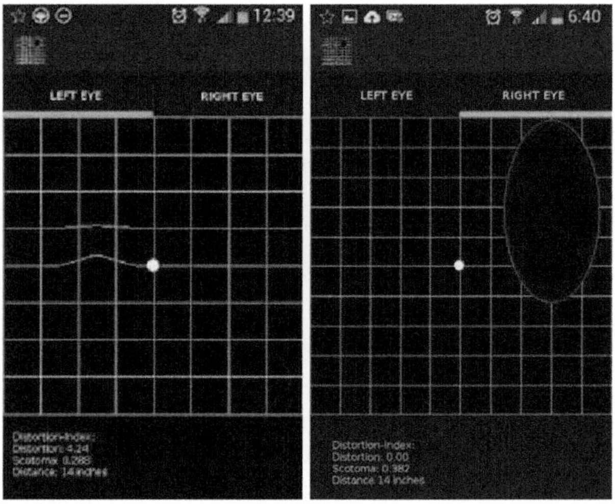

- ***Features***:

The app has been developed by Dr Ronald Krüger and offers a way to track the macular function of your AMD patients. The app was developed to measure degree, localization and area of distortions and visual field defects. It is based on the Amsler grid and implies the concept of a negative image: the patient has to straighten the lines that he monocularly sees distorted. The application reports indices represent amplitude, localization and area of distortions and are summarized in a sum index. There are also indices for area and localization of visual field defects in the application. The sensitivity of AMD application has been reported as 80% and specificity as 100% [2]. For wider range of pathologies, addition of the scotoma module in the app increased sensitivity from 0.84 to 0.94. Odds ratio to detect macular pathologies without metamorphopsias was 3.37: 95% CI, 0.94–5.67, when combining both app modules. The application can also be used to track improvement in AMD after anti-VEGF injections. It has been reported to show improvement in app indices that matches with decrease in macular thickness documented via OCT. The improvement also correlates with quality-of-life improvement as assessed by the National Eye Institute VFQ 25 scale [2]. Thus this application can be used as an effective real-world tool by AMD patients to assess improvement after interventions. The ability of the app to share this data in real time with the clinician further adds in to its potential use in teleophthalmology.

QR Scanning Code for the App

iOS Android

(e) ***Magnifier (Free)***

- ***Platforms***: iOS and Android
- ***App Creator***: TheSingularFactory
- ***Version***: 1.0.2
- ***App Size***: 45 MB
- ***App Icon***:

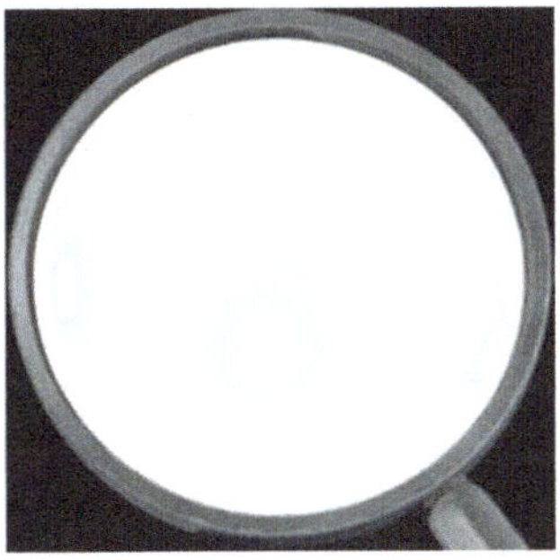

- ***App Screenshots***:

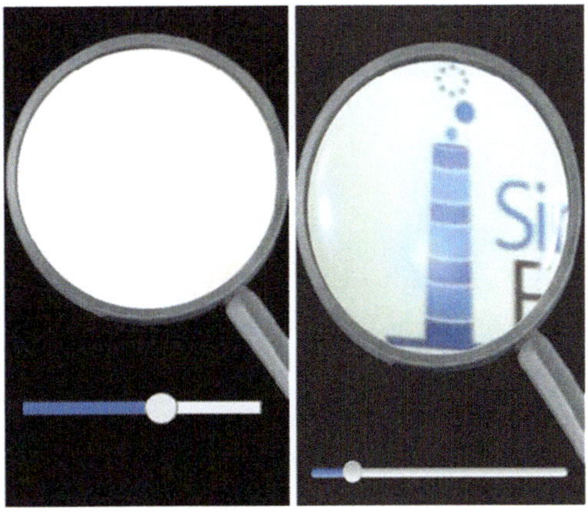

- ***Features***:
  The app has been developed by Juan José Flores Mederos to allow patients with presbyopia and ARMD to read small prints. With easy-to-use UI and clutter-free experience, this is one of the best applications that can aid these patients in everyday life.
  QR Scanning Code for the App

iOS

Android

(f) ***Ultra Magnifier (Free)***

- ***Platforms***: iOS
- ***App Creator***: zapDroid
- ***Version***: 1.8
- ***App Size***: 1.2 MB
- ***App Icon***:

- ***App Screenshots***:

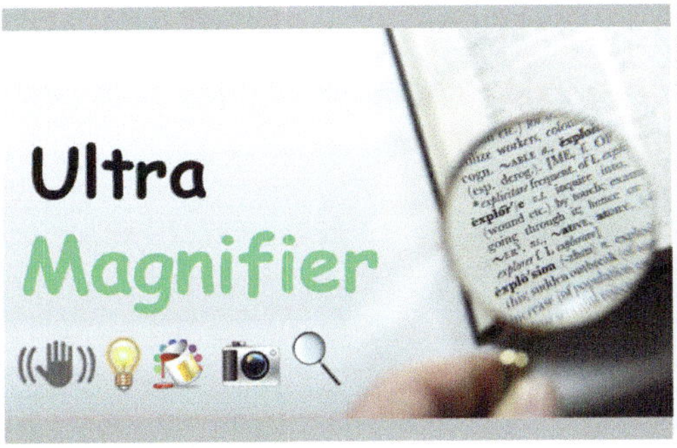

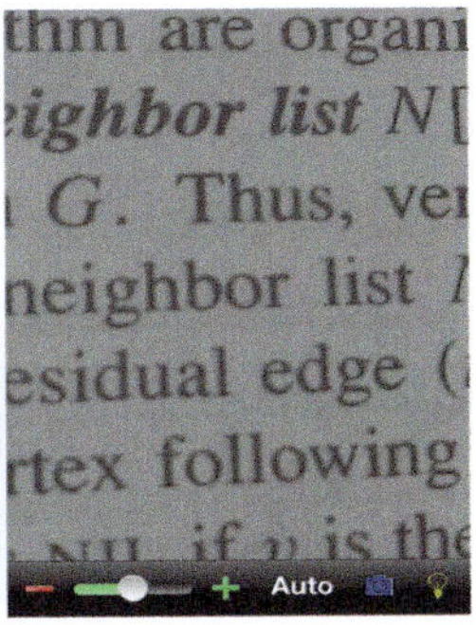

- ***Features***:
The app has been developed to be used as a pocket magnifying tool. The ability to use the autofocus function allows you to magnify and read small print and words. The patients can use the application to look at books, newspapers, restaurant's menu and receipts. The application can also be used in low light as it has a flashlight module as well.
QR Scanning Code for the App

2. **Diabetic Retinopathy**
   (a) ***Diabetic Retinopathy Predictor***
   - ***Platforms***: Android
   - ***App Creator***: David Folgado De la Rosa
   - ***Version***: 1.4
   - ***App Size***: 27 MB
   - ***App Icon***:

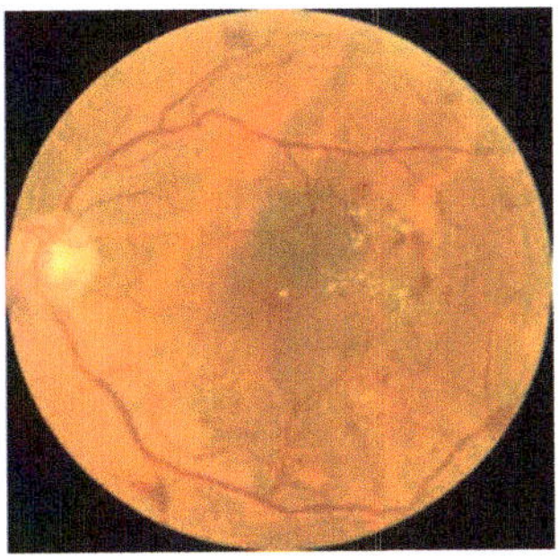

- ***App Screenshot***:

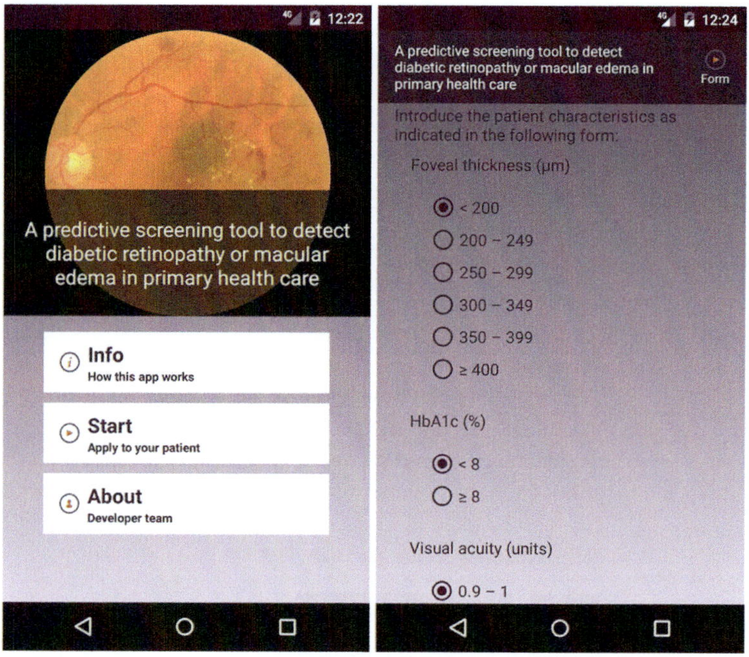

- ***Features***:

  This application is a medical calculator indicating the likelihood that a diabetic patient has diabetic retinopathy or not. The application requires glycosylated haemoglobin, HbA1c (%), foveal thickness (μm) and visual acuity (units), for calculation of a score. Patients with high HbA1c concentration, a greater foveal thickness and a lower visual acuity are at a higher risk of diabetic retinopathy. The results of the application can help a primary physician decide whether or not to refer the patient to a retina specialist. This application has been validated and gives promising results [3].

  QR Scanning Code for the App

(b) ***Diabetic Retinopathy***

- ***Platforms***: Android
- ***App Creator***: Focus Medica
- ***Version***: 1.0
- ***App Size***: 27 MB
- ***App Icon***:

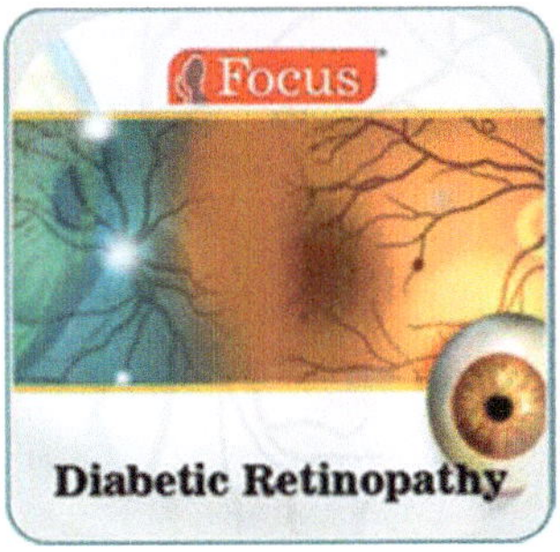

- ***App Screenshot***

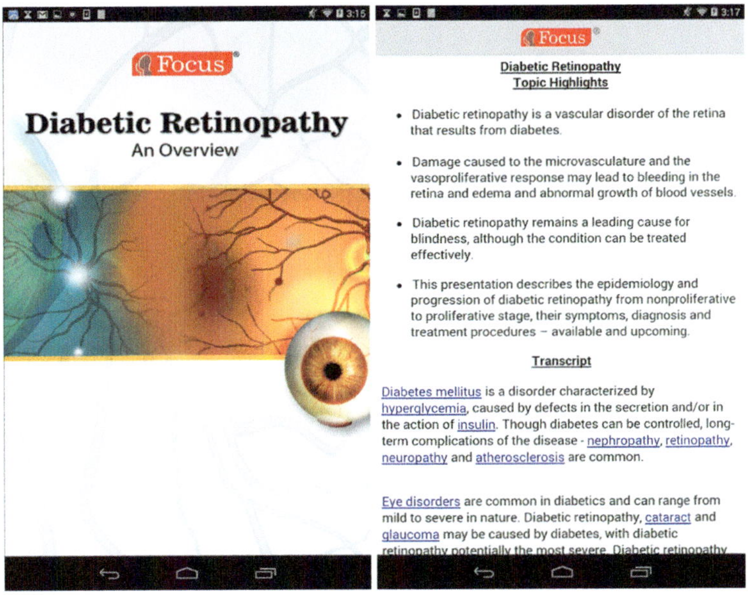

- ***Features***:

  This application discusses the epidemiology and pathophysiology of diabetic retinopathy including the risk factors, phases of disease progression, diagnostic tests, preventive guidelines and treatment options. It employs use of animated videos that can be easily understood by the patients as well.

QR Scanning Code for the App

3. **Retinopathy of Prematurity**
   (a) ***ROPQI***
   - ***Platforms***: Android
   - ***App Creator***: Deepak Chawla
   - ***Version***: 2.2
   - ***App Size***: 24.95 MB
   - ***App Icon***:

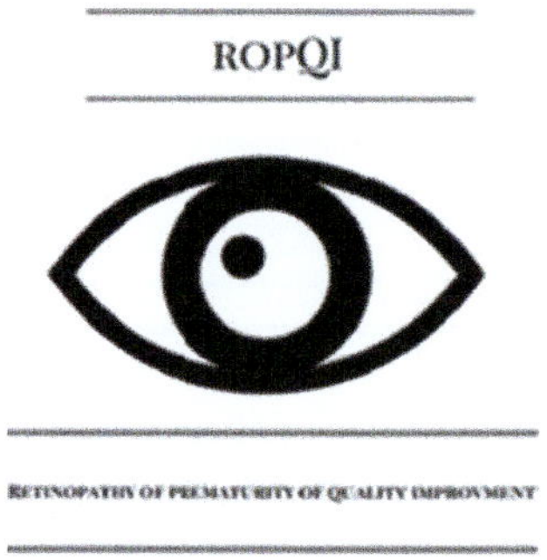

   - ***App Screenshot***:

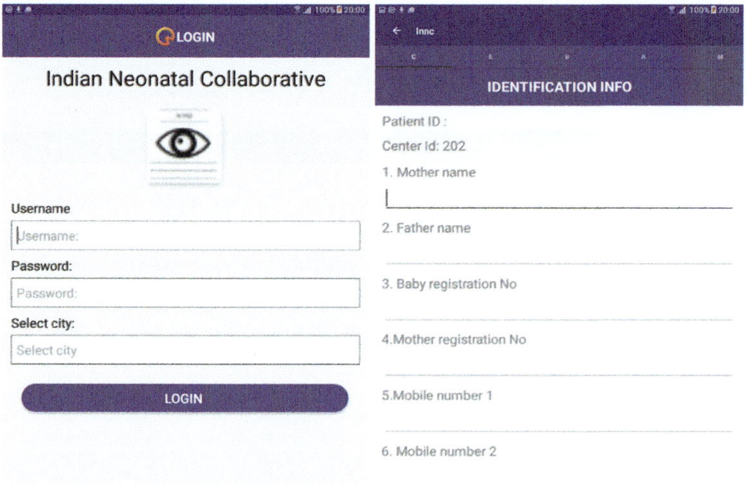

- ***Features***:
  This application is an aid to ROPQI (retinopathy of prematurity and quality improvement) programme. It can help paediatricians and ophthalmologists to store patient data. The application has an export option that can help create databases that can aid in better patient documentation.
  QR Scanning Code for the App

(b) ***iROP Assist***
- ***Platforms***: Android
- ***App Creator***: iROP Consortium
- ***Version***: 1.0.2
- ***App Size***: 18.82 MB
- ***App Icon***:

- ***App Screenshots***:

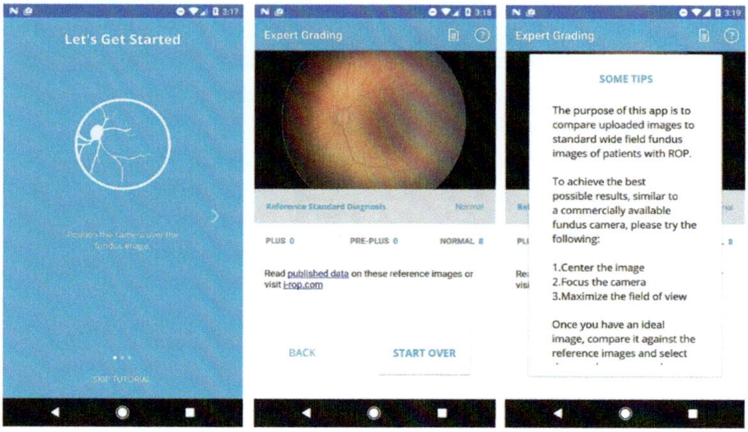

- ***Features***:
  This application is designed to allow clinicians to compare beside images of infants at risk for retinopathy of prematurity (ROP) with a published set of reference standard images. Users are able to upload fundus images and determine the relative severity of their image among the set of reference images by finding the image that most closely matches the relative degree of vascular abnormality. Published reference data for the spread of expert classifications (plus, pre-plus or normal) and reference standard diagnosis (consensus diagnosis of multiple independent image gradings and ophthalmoscopic diagnosis) is provided for the selected reference image.
  QR Scanning Code for the App

D. **Mobile Retinal Imaging**
Since the mobile technology boom, the quality of images that can be taken with mobile phones has surpassed all expectations. Several authors have described the use of this technology to take images of the eye. Simply using a condensing lens like 20D with a mobile phone can be effectively used to image the human retina. This was first reported by Bastawrous in 2012, and after that we have seen a boom in handheld fundus cameras or smart adaptors that can simplify the

otherwise tedious process [4]. From use for glaucoma, diabetes or ROP screening, mobile imaging technology is here to stay in ophthalmology [5–7]. The opportunity here is potentially limitless, and these devices will soon define patient screening at the primary level. Herein we describe some of the companion applications available to existing devices that are giving results comparable to tabletop expensive fundus cameras at fraction of their price [8].

1. ***Fundus-M***
   - ***Platforms***: iOS
   - ***App Creator***: Remidio Innovative Solutions Private Limited
   - ***Version***: 1.4
   - ***App Size***: 7.7 MB
   - ***App Icon***:

   - ***App Screenshots***:

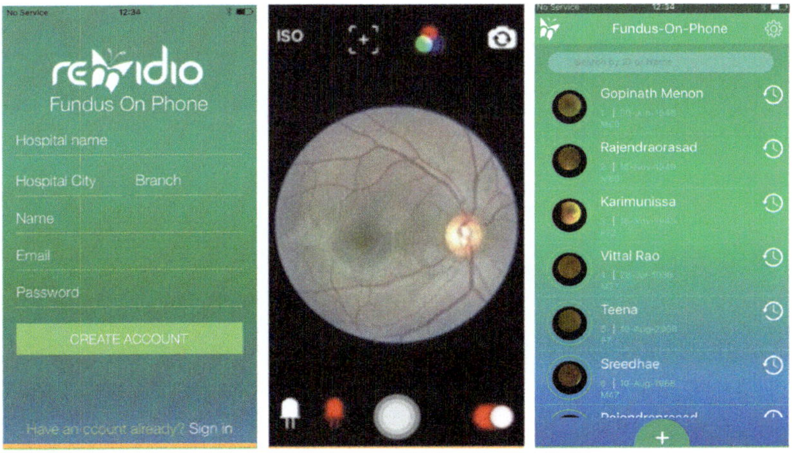

   - ***Features***:
     This application requires the Remidio Fundus on Phone (FOP) Device that can be purchased from QR code given below. It is available in a mydriatic and non-mydriatic model. The Fundus on Phone App can collect patient data in a searchable and sharable form. The metadata can be stamped on each image taken, enabling traceability of images. The app

also offers modest post-processing features like colour, tonal, sharpness, brightness and contrast and saturation changes. Recently they have added the Wi-Fi-direct capability to allow wireless printing of the images.

The device has been compared to a Zeiss camera in a study of 602 eyes. The sensitivity and specificity for detecting any DR by FOP were 92.7% and 98.4%, respectively, with the Zeiss camera, and the kappa (κ) agreement was 0.90, while for PDR with macular oedema, the sensitivity was 87.9%, specificity was 94.9%, and κ agreement was 0.80, compared to conventional photography [9].

QR Scanning Code for the App and the Website

App Website (Buy FOP)

2. ***MII Ret Cam***
   - ***Platforms***: Android (Free Trial) and iOS (44.99$ for Pro Version)
   - ***App Creator***: Dr Ashish Sharma
   - ***Version***: 1.0.5 (Android), 2.1(iOS)
   - ***App Size***: 3.20 MB(Android), 15.8 MB(Android)
   - ***App Icon***:

- ***App Screenshots***:

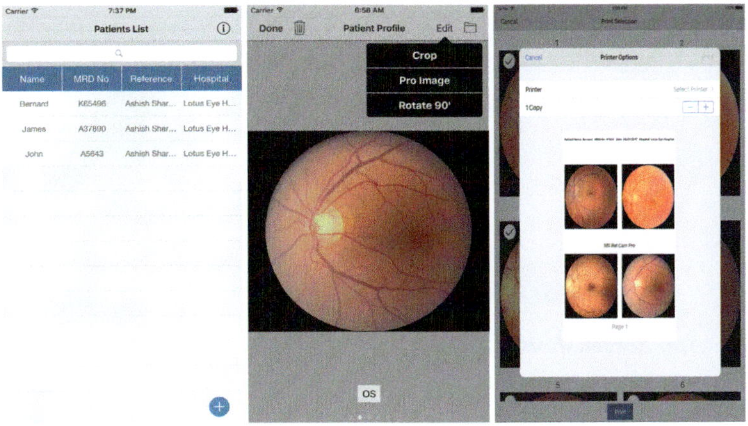

- ***Features***:

  MII Ret Cam app is a patient management tool which is designed for doctors to capture patient's details along with images/documents using the MII Ret Cam adaptor that can be purchased using the below given QR code. The UI design is elegant and simple. The app allows live view of the fundus, tagging of images and seamless sharing capabilities. The iOS version also allows control of the camera LED brightness. The pro mode additionally offers the pro picture filter that transforms the mobile images into cropped versions that look similar to images taken from any tabletop fundus camera. The MII Ret Cam is available for 19,999 INR and 380 USD. You can also find the instruction videos using the QR code given below.

  QR Scanning Code for the App

  Android iOS Website (Buy) Youtube

3. ***oDocs Capture***
   - ***Platforms***: iOS
   - ***App Creator***: Sheng Chiong Hong
   - ***Version***: 1.0
   - ***App Size***: 14.80 MB

- ***App Icon***:

- ***App Screenshots***:

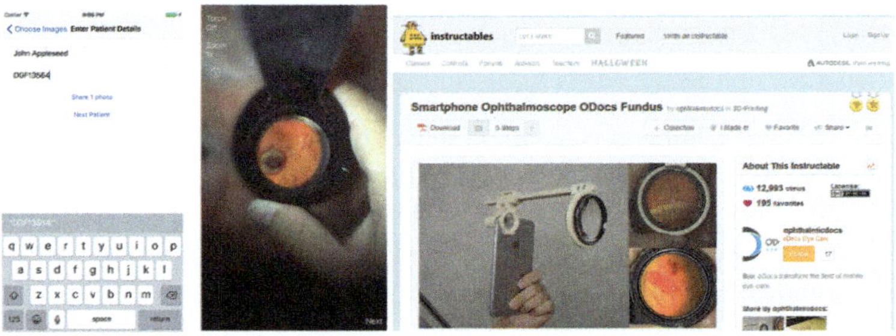

- ***Features***:

  3D printing is still uncharted territory for the uninitiated in mobile technology. However the potential that 3D printing has is being unearthed every day. The 3D-printed oDocs Retina Adaptor is freely available to all [10]. It can be printed at home under 50$. The device can also be bought preprinted and assembled from the QR link given below. This companion application allows the doctor to take anterior segment and retinal images using oDocs devices. The app helps in capturing images with one-handed controls and has a streamlined interface. The images can also be quickly exported to your computer or the cloud for storage. The application also lets you share the images with colleagues to facilitate faster analysis.

  QR Scanning Code for the App

iOS Website (Buy) Instructable Link

These ***companion*** applications however require adaptors that are costly. The quality of images obtained and the feature-rich interface of the applications justify the cost; still options are available for the DIY enthusiasts to fashion their own mobile imaging devices. Links to some of them are given below:

- The 20 D technique: doi: 10.1016/j.ophtha.2011.11.014
- The Raspberry Pi Device: doi: 10.1155/2017/4526243
- DIY Ret CAM: http://www.ijo.in/text.asp?2016/64/9/663/194325

4. ***OCT Browser***
   - ***Platforms***: iPad
   - ***App Creator***: Hiroshi Ishikawa
   - ***Version***: 1.0
   - ***App Size***: 57.4 MB
   - ***App Icon***:

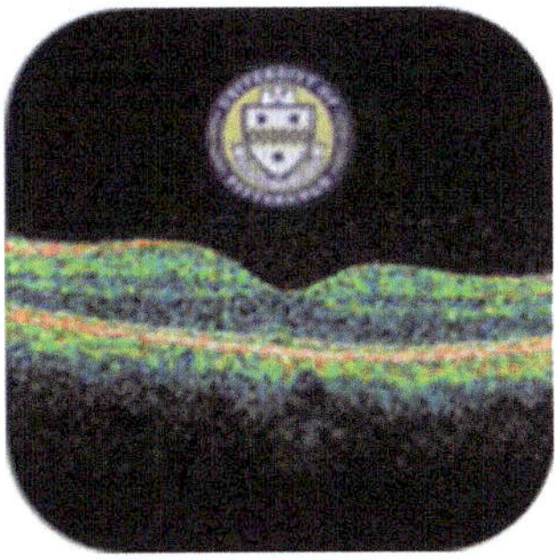

   - ***App Screenshots***:

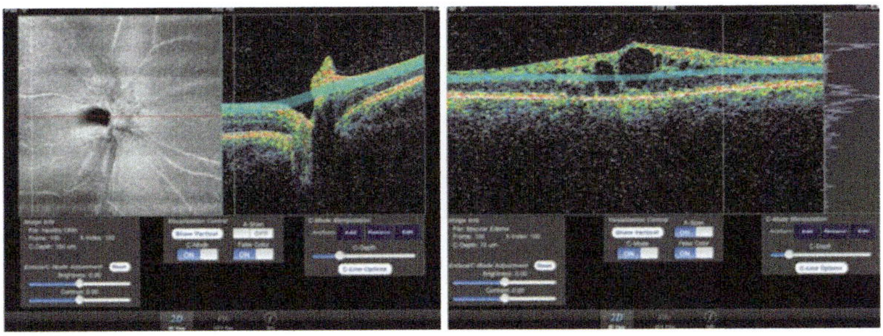

   - ***Features***:

     This app is a part of OCT Browser Software Suite. Retina specialists usually have to review piles of still images. It is time-consuming to directly manipulate images, sitting in front of the OCT machine during busy clinics. As soon as an OCT scan is done, 3D OCT images can be converted to an iPad-friendly portable format and delivered to the doctor's iPad. This eases the scan reviews by the doctor. The app has speckle noise reduction and signal optimization function. The images can be shared with colleagues and the patient.

QR Scanning Code for the App

Social Networking for Vitreoretina

A. ***Web Resources***

1. ***ASRS***: The American Society of Retina Specialists is the largest retinal organization in the world, with nearly 3000 members in the USA and 59 countries. ASRS provides variety of educational resources to help physicians expand their knowledge and abilities to diagnose and treat vitreoretinal diseases with the most advanced concepts and techniques available. The educational resources include Retina Times, CME's, Spotlight cases, Retina Image Bank, schedule of ASRS meetings, etc.

   Website Screenshots

   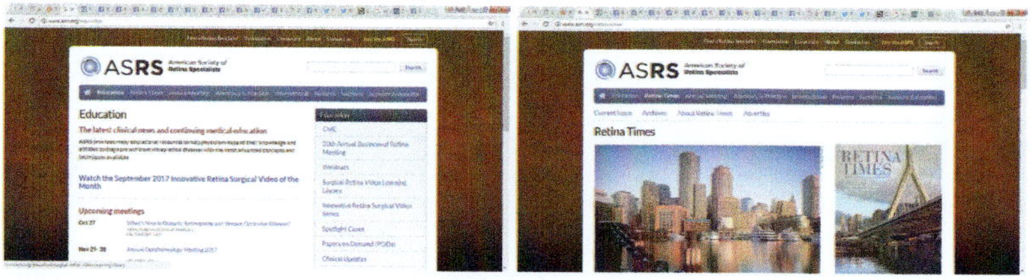

   Site URL: ***http://www.asrs.org/home***

2. ***The Retina Society***: The Retina Society began as an extension of alumni meetings of the Retina Associates, a retina practice founded in Boston in 1951 by Charles L. Schepens. The society strives to reduce worldwide visual disability and blindness by promoting the education and professional interaction of vitreoretinal specialists as well as providing optimal care for patients with vitreoretinal diseases. Basic and clinical research are encouraged to further patient care.

Website Screenshots

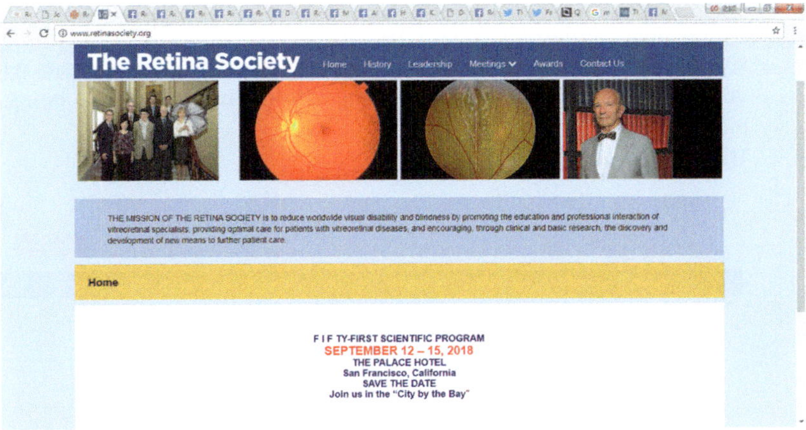

Site URL*: *http://www.retinasociety.org/

3. ***The Macula Society***: The Macula Society is a forum for latest research for retinal, vascular and macular diseases. Membership is by application, with acceptance criteria including extensive contribution to retinal literature. The Macula Society recognizes outstanding achievement by its members and others through awards and lectures.
Website Screenshots

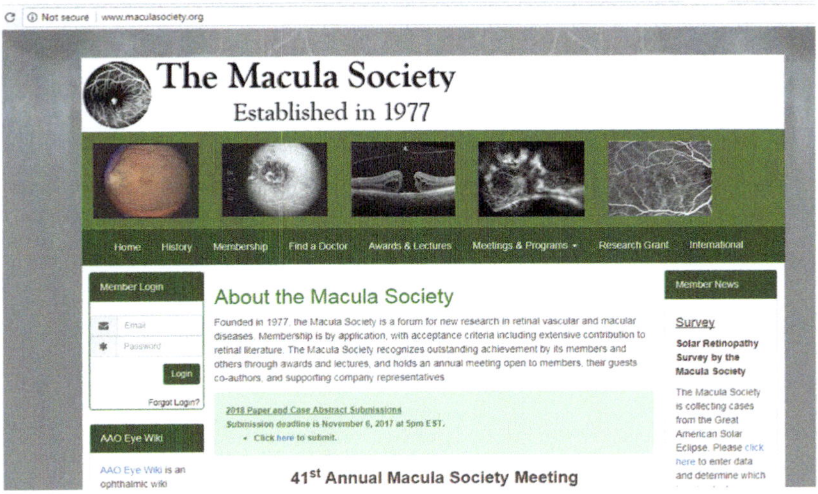

Site URL*: *http://www.maculasociety.org

4. ***Vitreo Retinal Society of India***: The Vitreo Retina Society of India (VRSI) was founded in 1992, by a small group of 20 vitreoretinal specialists under the presidentship of Dr. T. N. Ursekar and Dr. Rumi P. Jahangir. This exclusive group has now expanded to over 300 vitreoretinal specialists with over 90% of the India's actively practicing vitreoretinal specialists being its life members.
Website Screenshots

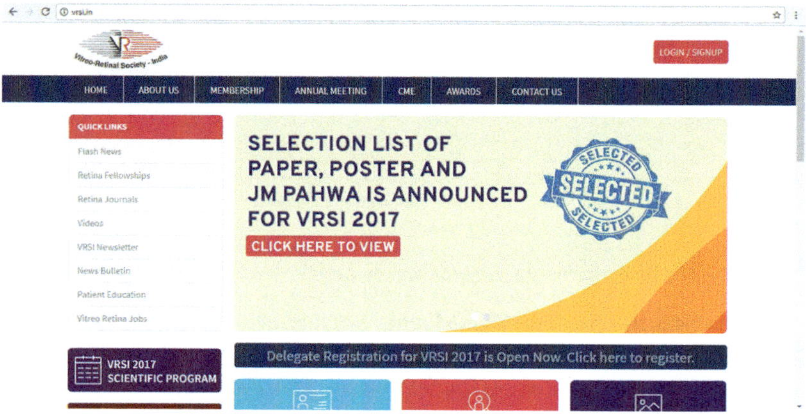

Site URL: ***http://vrsi.in/***

5. ***RetNet***: RetNet, Retinal Information Network, is a source of knowing the genes and loci causing inherited retinal diseases, such as retinitis pigmentosa, macular degeneration and Usher syndrome. This information is provided to the research community and other interested individuals for research purposes only.
Website Screenshots

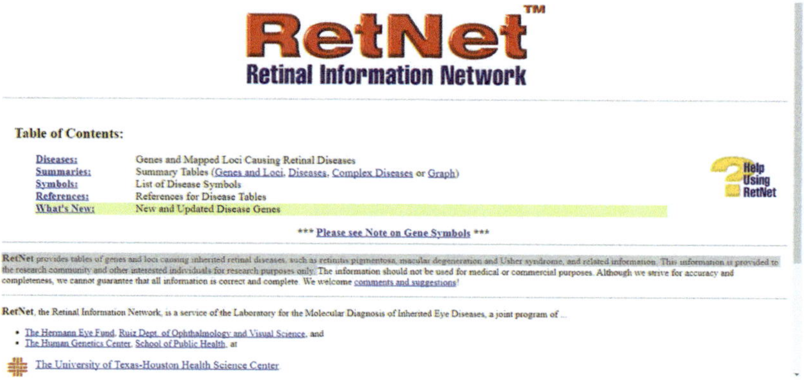

Site URL: ***https://sph.uth.edu/retnet/***

B. ***Facebook Pages***

S. No	Page icon	Page name	Description	QR code
Retina society pages				
1.		EURETINA	The European Society of Retina Specialists (EURETINA) is Europe's largest society of retina specialists. The society currently has 1000 members across over 90 countries	
2.		Macular Society	The Macular Society is a charity for anyone affected by central vision loss. This society has the largest membership group in the sight loss sector and the voice of people with macular conditions	
Journal pages				
1.		Retina	Official page of the Retina journal	
2.		Retina Today	Official page of Retina Today	

S. No	Page icon	Page name	Description	QR code
Physician information and training				
1.	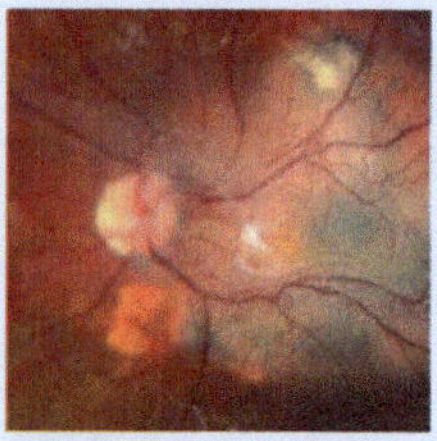	Retina	This page is dedicated to all the vitreoretinal specialist and retinal enthusiast who share personal experiences and knowledge via this platform	
2.	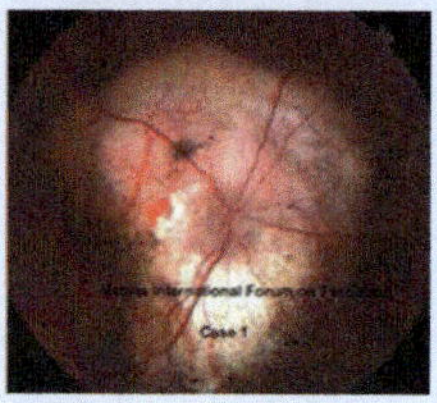	Retina International Forum	Another community page that offers regular updates from the subspeciality	
Patient support groups				
1.		Retina India	Retina India is a not-for-profit organization established for empowering people with retinal disorders and for those with an interest in retinal diseases	
2.		Retina Foundation	A commercial page but has excellent images and patient information posts	
3.		Retina Australia	Official page of Retina Australia	

S. No	Page icon	Page name	Description	QR code
Disease-specific pages				
1.		Macular Degeneration Research	Macular Degeneration Research (MDR), a programme of BrightFocus Foundation, funds research on and informs the public about macular degeneration	
2.	AMDF	American Macular Degeneration Foundation	The American Macular Degeneration Foundation works for the prevention, treatment and cure of macular degeneration through raising funds, educating the public and supporting scientific research	
3.	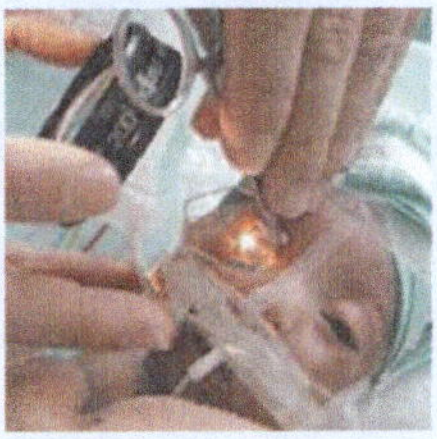	HOPE for ROP	This page publishes and receives articles and news related to stem cell treatment research that can bring HOPE for children and adults that are struggling for treatments that could heal ROP	
4.	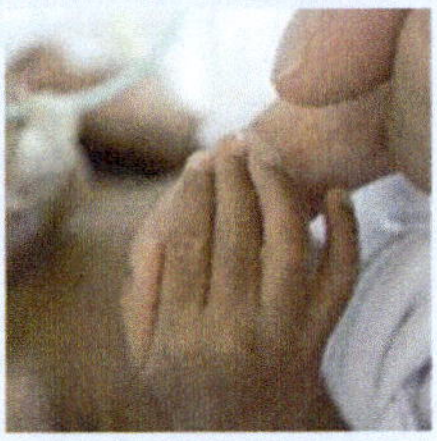	KIDROP	Brainchild of Dr Anand Vinekar, KIDROP uses teleophthalmology since 2008 to screen for ROP in unreached rural areas. In 2010, it became the largest Tele-ROP network in the world	
5.	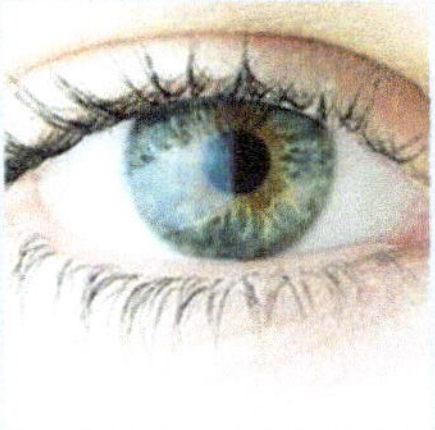	Retinitis Pigmentosa Community Support	A community support group for patients with retinitis pigmentosa	

C. ***Twitter Handles***

S. No	Handle icon	Handle name	Description	QR code
1.	EURETINA European Society of Retina Specialists	EURETINA	Official account of EURETINA	
2.	RT	Retina Today	Official account of Retina Today	
3.	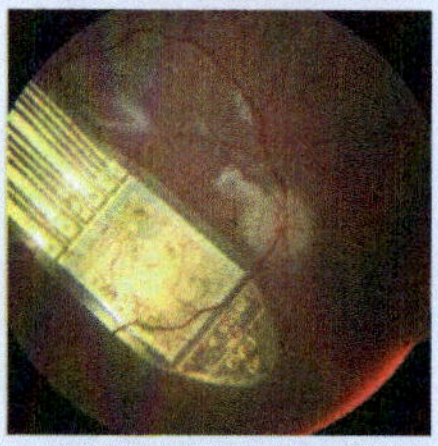	Retina Implant	Official account of Retina Implant AG	
4.	NRMD	New Retina MD	Official account of New Retina MD	
5.	RetinaCME	RetinaCME	Official account of Retina CME	

S. No	Handle icon	Handle name	Description	QR code
6.	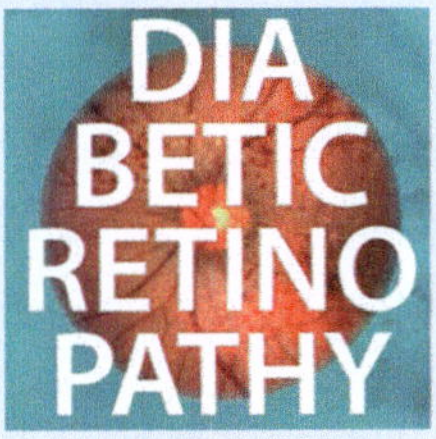	Diabetic Eyes	The account regularly posts information about diabetes and how it affects the eyes	
7.	THE RETINITIS PIGMENTOSA COMMUNITY	TheRPCommunity	This is a support group for patients with retinitis pigmentosa	

Applications for Uveal Diseases

Uveal diseases most often transcend the borders between medicine and ophthalmology. There are a few resources that can help you formulate a diagnosis without having to order a battery of investigations.

1. ***Uveitis Doctor (2.99$)***
    - ***Platforms***: iOS
    - ***App Creator***: Javier Lara Medina
    - ***Version***: 2.1 iOS
    - ***App Size***: 91.9 MB
    - ***App Icon***:

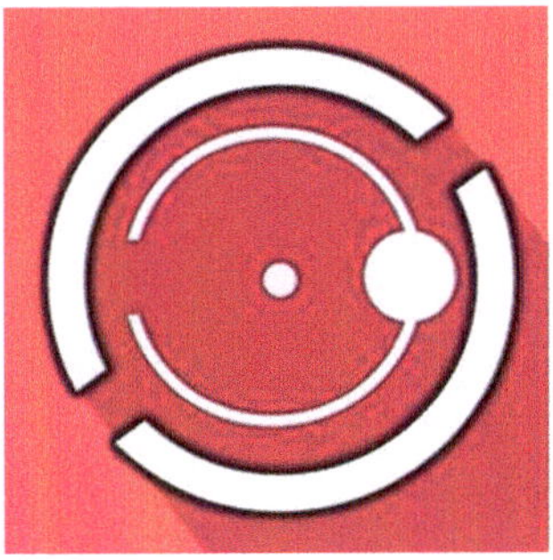

- ***App Screenshots***:

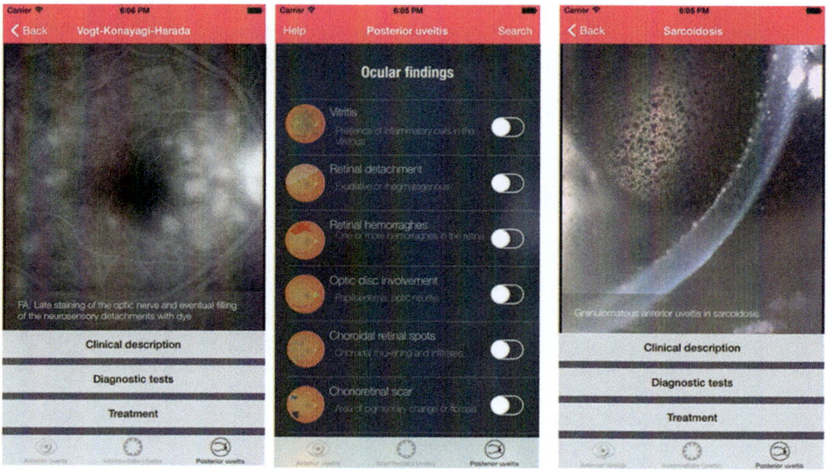

- ***Features***:
  This application is capable of making the differential diagnosis of more than 100 types of uveitis based on a few details of the history or ocular findings. The application has a database organized according to the location of the inflammation and includes multiple descriptive data for each of the diseases. The database includes hundreds of diagnostic possibilities, including a description of the pathology, diagnostic tests needed to complete the diagnosis (for naming and meshing) and potential treatment strategy. The app also has a photographic atlas of uveitis that can be used for referencing.
  QR Scanning Codes for the App

2. ***Uvemaster ($14.99)***
   - ***Platforms***: iOS and Android
   - ***App Creator***: Leading Smart Health Technology
   - ***Version***: 2.61 Android
   - ***App Size***: 91.9 MB
   - ***App Icon***:

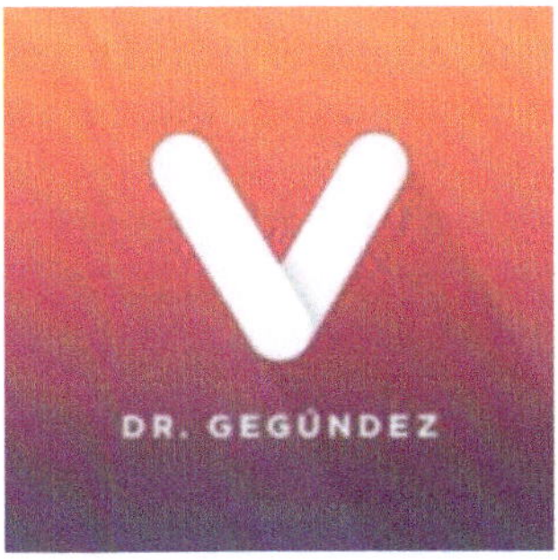

   - ***App Screenshots***:

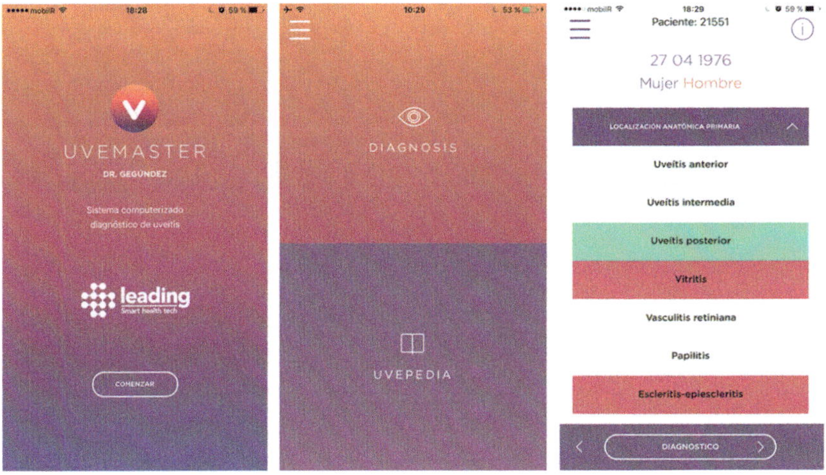

- ***Features***:
  This application is a computer-assisted system to diagnose uveitis, developed by Dr. José Antonio Gegúndez Fernández. Uvemaster has a mathematical algorithm by which any doctor can make a differential diagnosis approach to a patient with uveitis. The user only has to mark the clinical signs, both present and absent, according to the defined criteria. The app contains a large database of 88 uveitis syndromes each with 76 clinical items, both ocular and systemic (total 6688), and displays a differential diagnoses list (DDL) ordered by sensitivity, specificity or positive predictive value (PPV). The app has been validated and has a high diagnostic accuracy (96.6%). By sensitivity, the original diagnosis appeared among the top three in the DDL in 90.9% and was the first in 73.9%. Considering the PPV, the original diagnosis was among the top DDL three in 62.5% and the first in 29.5% [11]. This suggests that the app can thus may become a reliable tool for an ophthalmologist.
  QR Scanning Codes for the App

  Android

  iOS

Social Networking For Uvea

A. ***Web Resources***
   1. ***Diagnose Uveitis***: This online tool offers the ability to formulate a diagnosis on the basis of clinical findings that are present in your patient. The website is free to use and has an engaging user interface.

Website Screenshots

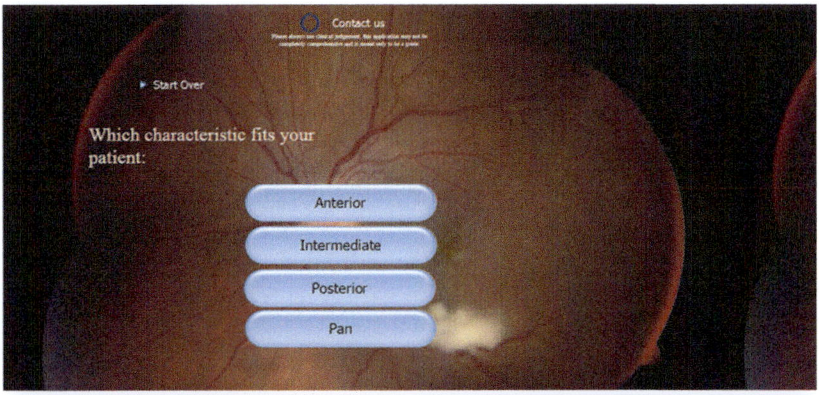

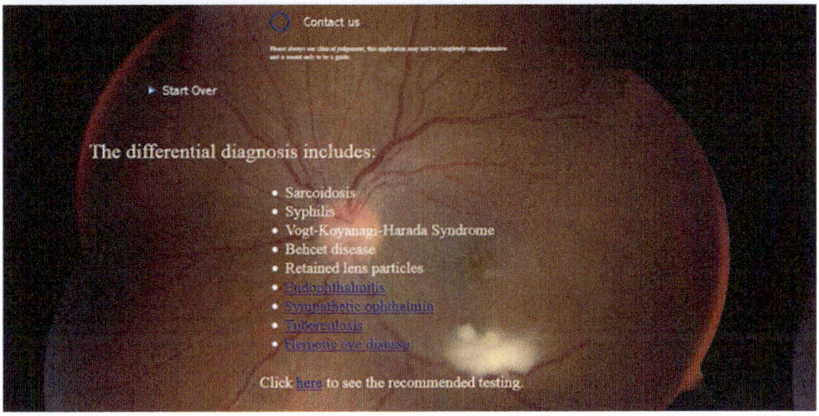

***Site URL**: http://www.diagnoseuveitis.com/default.html*

2. ***Olivia Vision***: This website was established in 2010 to provide information, support and advice for anyone affected by uveitis.
Website Screenshots

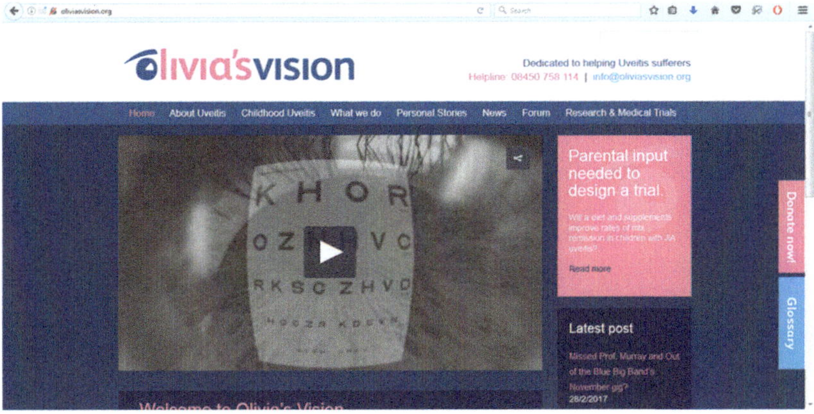

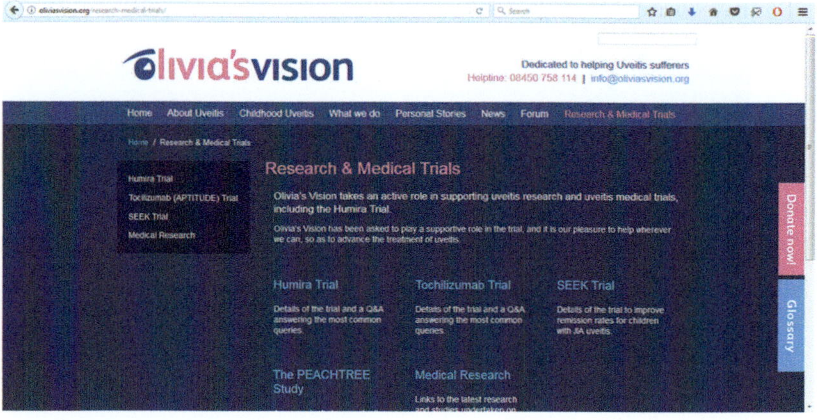

***Site URL**: http://oliviasvision.org/*

3. ***American Uveitis Society***: Since 1990, the American Uveitis Society is functional as an educational, non-profit corporation. The main objective of the society is to increase knowledge regarding uveitis in the medical and research professions through instructional courses, clinics, lectures and seminars, at which members and renowned speakers present subjects of current interest and relevance. The website keeps the physician members updated about the society's day-to-day activities.
   Website Screenshots

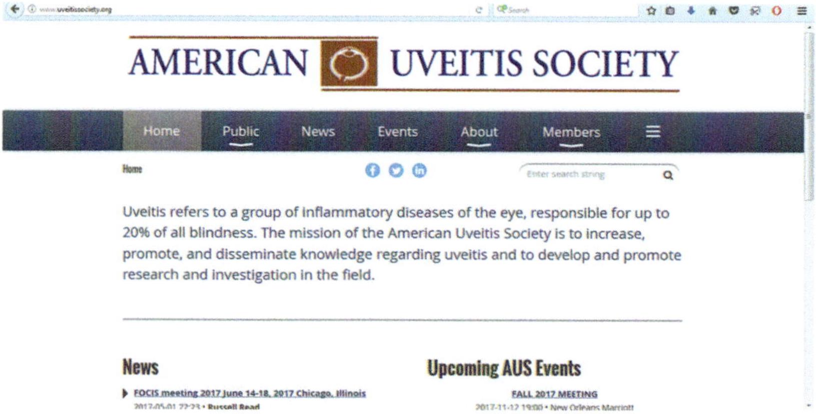

***Site URL**: http://www.uveitissociety.org/*

B. ***Facebook Pages***

S. No	Page icon	Page name	Description	QR code
Uveitis related pages				
1.	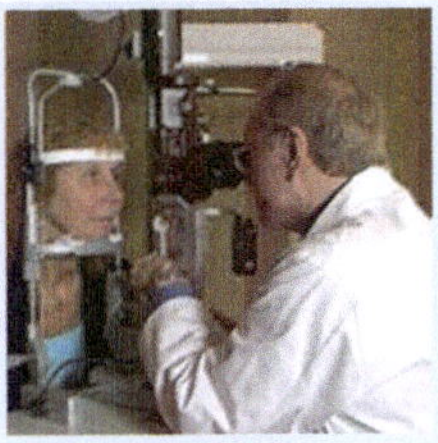	Uveitis	Official page of the MERSI Uveitis group. Keeps you updated about uveitis	
2.	Uveitis Patient Support Group	Uveitis Patient Support Group @UPGSonline	Official page of the Uveitis Patient Support Group	
3.	USI	Uveitis Society of India @uveitissocietyofindia	Official page of the Uveitis Society of India	

C. ***Twitter Handles***

S. No	Handle icon	Handle name	Description	QR code
1.	BIRDSHOT CHORIORETINOPATHY UVEITIS SOCIETY	Birdshot Charity	Official handle of the Birdshot Charity	
2.	OIUF THE OCULAR IMMUNOLOGY AND UVEITIS FOUNDATION Dedicated to Eye Disease Cure and Education	Uveitis1	Official handle of the OIUF	

S. No	Handle icon	Handle name	Description	QR code
3.		Olivia's Vision	Official handle of the Uveitis Charity	

References

1. Agarwal A, Afridi R, Agrawal R, Do DV, Gupta V, Nguyen QD. Multimodal imaging in retinal vasculitis. Ocul Immunol Inflamm. 2017;25(3):424–33.
2. Claessens D, Krüger RV. AMD - a metamorphopsia detector. Invest Ophthalmol Vis Sci. 2015;56(7):4109.
3. Azrak C, Palazon-Bru A, Baeza-Diaz MV, Folgado-De la Rosa DM, Hernandez-Martinez C, Martinez-Toldos JJ, et al. A predictive screening tool to detect diabetic retinopathy or macular edema in primary health care: construction, validation and implementation on a mobile application. Peer J. 2015;e1404:3.
4. Bastawrous A. Smartphone fundoscopy. Ophthalmology. 2012;119(2):432–3.e2.
5. Ryan ME, Rajalakshmi R, Prathiba V, Anjana RM, Ranjani H, Narayan KMV, et al. Comparison Among Methods of Retinopathy Assessment (CAMRA) study: smartphone, nonmydriatic, and mydriatic photography. Ophthalmology. 2015;122(10):2038–43.
6. Bastawrous A, Giardini ME, Bolster NM, Peto T, Shah N, Livingstone IA, et al. Clinical validation of a smartphone-based adapter for optic disc imaging in Kenya. JAMA Ophthalmol. 2016;134(2):151–8.
7. Furdova A, Furdova A, Krcmery V. Our experience with smartphone and spherical lens for the eye fundus examination during humanitarian project in Africa. Int J Ophthalmol. 2017;10(1):157–60.
8. Jin K, Lu H, Su Z, Cheng C, Ye J, Qian D. Telemedicine screening of retinal diseases with a handheld portable non-mydriatic fundus camera. BMC Ophthalmol. 2017;17(1):89.
9. Rajalakshmi R, Arulmalar S, Usha M, Prathiba V, Kareemuddin KS, Anjana RM, et al. Validation of smartphone based retinal photography for diabetic retinopathy screening. PLoS One. 2015;10(9):e0138285.
10. Hong SC. 3D printable retinal imaging adapter for smartphones could go global. Graefes Arch Clin Exp Ophthalmol. 2015;253(10):1831–3.
11. Gegundez-Fernandez JA, Fernandez-Vigo JI, Diaz-Valle D, Mendez-Fernandez R, Cuina-Sardina R, Santos-Bueso E, et al. Uvemaster: a mobile app-based decision support system for the differential diagnosis of uveitis. Invest Ophthalmol Vis Sci. 2017;58(10):3931–9.

Apps and Social Networking Pages for Corneal Disorders

6

Cornea is no longer considered a single 0.5 mm of clear tissue, but as a layered structure. Better recognition and diagnosis of corneal disorders and advent of newer procedures such as collagen crosslinking, intracorneal implants, anterior lamellar keratoplasty, endothelial keratoplasty and femtosecond laser refractive surgery have changed the traditional approach to managing corneal disorders.

Apps listed in this chapter would help cornea specialists, comprehensive ophthalmologists and allied health personnel who are actively managing patients with important diseases of the cornea and ocular surface.

Applications

The apps are discussed under the following sections:

A. Apps for contact lenses
B. Apps for keratoconus
C. Apps for ocular surface
D. Apps for refractive surgery

A. **Apps for Contact Lenses**
   Apps for Ophthalmologists and Optometrists
   1. **CL Calcs**
      - ***Platforms***: iPhone, iPad, iPod Touch ($4.99)
      - ***App Creator***: Todd Zarwell
      - ***Version***: 1.13
      - ***App Size***: 4.3 MB

P. Ichhpujani, S. Thakur, *Smart Resources in Ophthalmology*, Current Practices in Ophthalmology, https://doi.org/10.1007/978-981-13-0140-7_6

- ***App Icon***:

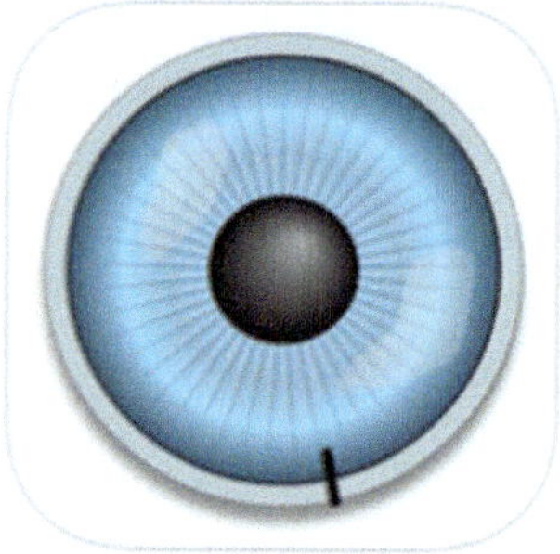

- ***App Screenshot***:

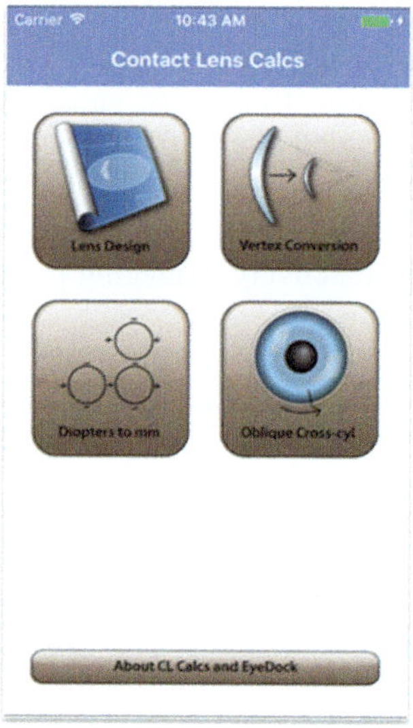

- ***Features***:

  The CL Calcs app has a vertexing calculator to convert a spectacle prescription to the corneal plane. It accepts and returns results in plus or minus cylinder and allows for different vertex distances.

  Additionally, the app has vertexing tables, an oblique cross-cylinder calculator, keratometry conversion calculator and keratometry conversion tables.

  It suggests the appropriate contact lens design and gives pros and cons of the available options, for example, bitoric versus back toric.

QR Scanning Code for the App

2. **Optical Contact Lens Calculator**
   - ***Platforms***: iOS (iPhone and iPad)
   - ***App Creator***: Rob McQualter
   - ***Version***: 1.9
   - ***App Size***: 7.8 MB
   - ***App Icon***:

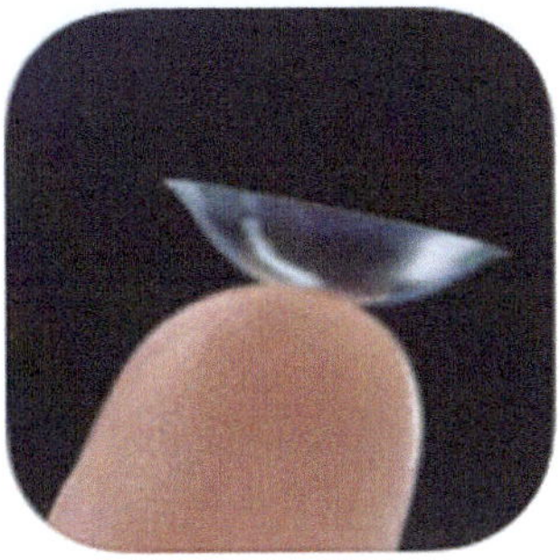

- ***App Screenshots***:

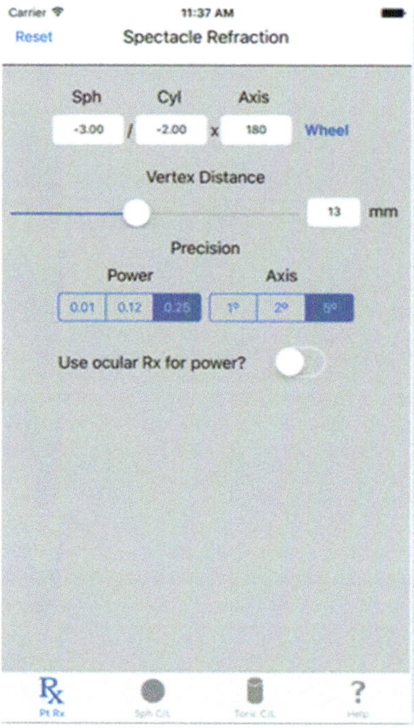

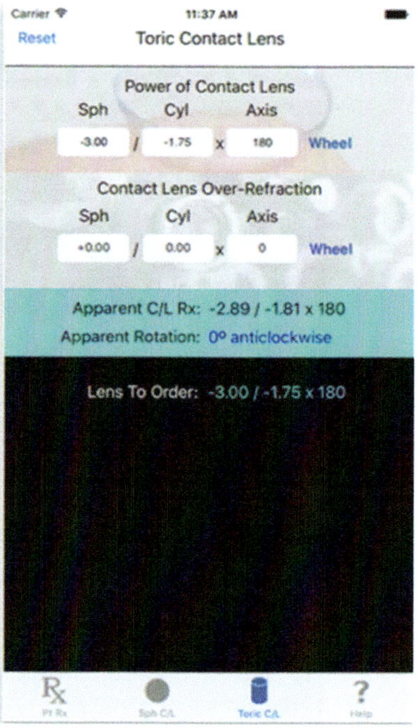

- ***Features***:

Opticalc Contact Lens Calculator is a helpful tool for fitting of soft contact lenses. This app uses patient's refraction and vertex distance to calculate the ocular refraction corrected for vertex distance and provides a recommended spherical contact lens power based on the patient's spherocylindrical refraction.

If the toric contact lens is mislocating, the app can tell by how much the lens is mislocating and suggest a new lens to order.

Using the power of the patient's contact lens and the spectacle over-refraction, Opticalc can tell the amount of lens rotation (degrees) and recommend the correct lens power. This app may also help to minimize the number of reorders required for toric patients and make the initial lens selection for spherical patients more precise.

QR Scanning Code for the App

3. **Contact Lens Toric Eye App**
   - ***Platforms***: Android and iOS
   - ***App Creator***: Bausch and Lomb
   - ***Version***: 2.0
   - ***App Size***: 19.6 MB
   - ***App Icon***:

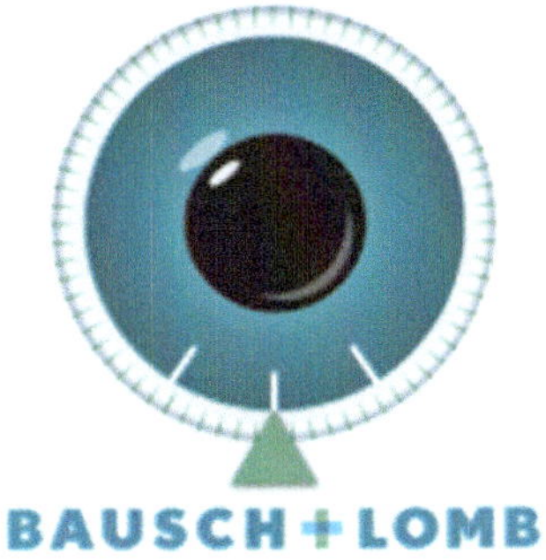

   - ***App Screenshots***:

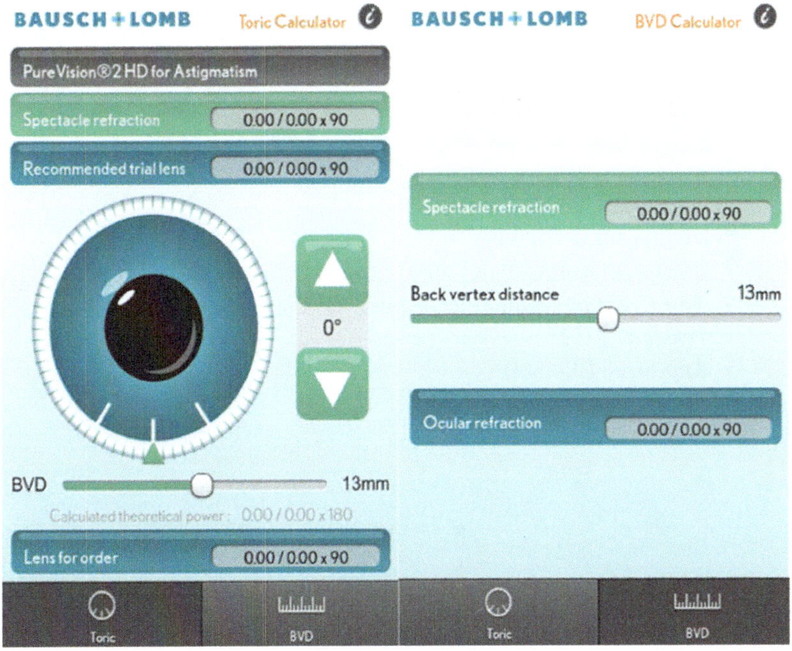

- ***Features***:
  This free application helps to calculate which toric contact lens is appropriate for a specific astigmatic prescription. Using industry standard calculations, the app calculates what initial trial lens should be used with a given spectacle prescription. If after fitting the lens rotates off axis, the tool calculates the new axis direction for lens trial. The app uses an image depicting a toric lens with axis markings that the user can rotate on screen. The app also offers an over-refraction calculator.

  Additionally, for prescriptions over ±5.00 dioptres in either meridians, a back vertex calculator is added in to calculate the power required for those prescriptions. This toric calculator tool supplies both the calculated theoretical power for use with any manufacturer's lenses and specific parameters for Bausch + Lomb toric lens portfolio.

  QR Scanning Code for the App

  iOS Android

4. **Eye Calculator**: **(0.99$)**
   - ***Platform***: Android and iOS
   - ***App Creator***: Manuel Rodriguez Vallejo
   - ***Version***: 1.0.2
   - ***App Size***: 13.4 MB
   - ***App Icon***:

- ***App Screenshots***:

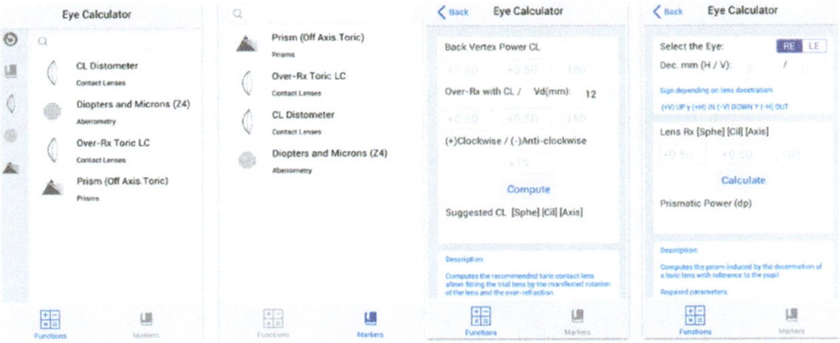

- ***Features***:
  This app checks distometry with contact lenses, converts diopters to micras (and vice versa) for defocus aberration, computes the final toric contact lens after over-refraction and checks for prismatic effect induced by a toric lens decentration.

  QR Scanning Code for the App

  iOS Android

5. **Crossed-Cylinder Calculator**
   - ***Platforms***: iOS (iPhone and iPad)
   - ***App Creator***: Alta Vista LLC
   - ***Version***: 1.1

- ***App Size***: 9 MB
- ***App Icon***:

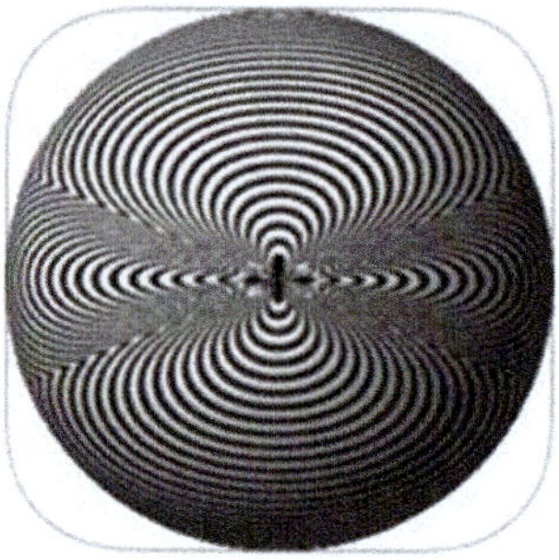

- ***App Screenshots***:

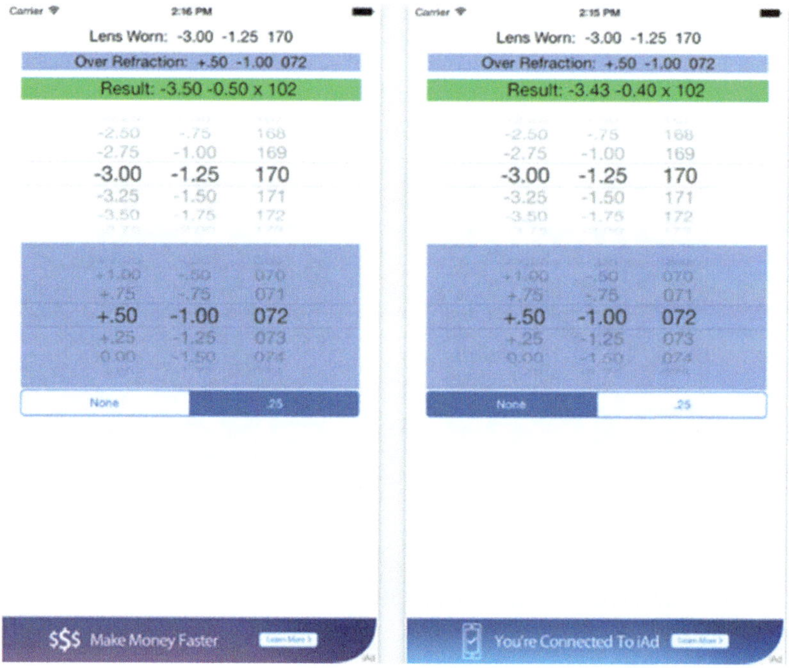

- ***Features***:
  This app helps to determine resultant lens over existing lens combined with over-refraction. This increases the accuracy of the contact lens fitting and helps in refining high powered eyeglass prescriptions using over-refraction. Resulting contact lens prescription or spectacle prescription can also be determined using lens currently worn and over-refraction data.

QR Scanning Code for the App

- ***Apps for Contact Lens Wearers***
  People use contact lenses either for therapeutic or cosmetic reasons. One of the most common problems with contact lenses is that the patients don't change their contact lenses on time, simply because they forget. They just don't remember to change them after 14 or 30 days. For such patients reminder apps are really helpful. This section enlists some of them.

1. **Contact Lens Tracker**
   - ***Platforms***: iOS (iPhone and iPad)
   - ***App Creator***: Stuart Radforth
   - ***Version***: 3.0.0
   - ***App Size***: 11.1 MB
   - ***App Icon***:

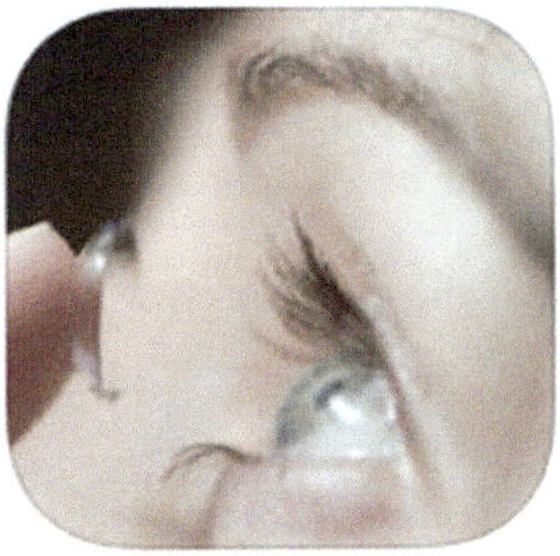

- ***App Screenshot***:

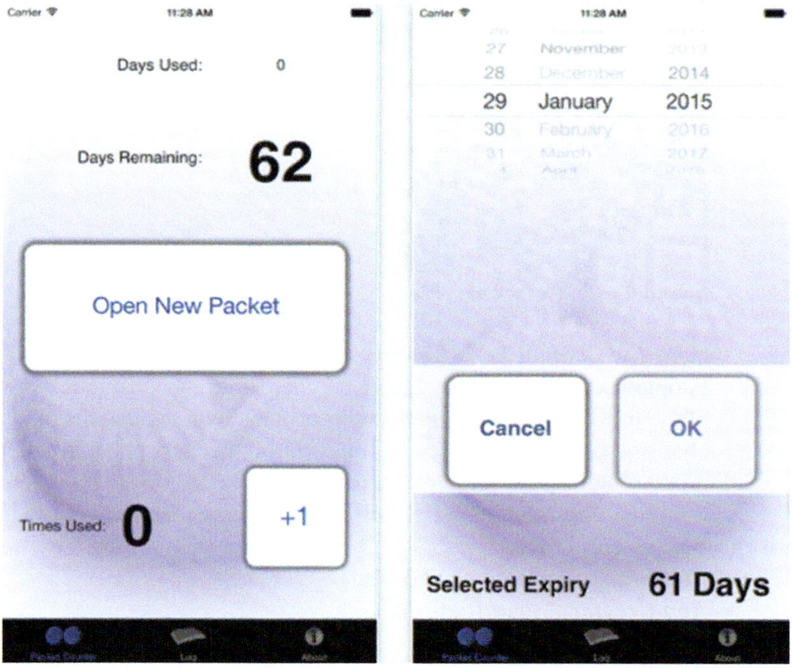

- ***Features***:
  This app helps the user to keep a track of their reusable contact lenses. The user needs to press the 'Open Packet' button when they start a new set of reusable lenses and specify the due date of expiry for the pack (from 1 to 366 days). Once a pack is opened, the user needs to press the '+1' button to increment the count.

  There is a history tab to see the date when the packet was opened and how many times that packet was used (along with dates of usages).

  QR Scanning Code for the App

2. **EyeMinder Contact Lens Reminder**
    - ***Platform***: Android and iOS
    - ***App Creator***: OPHTHALMX, LLC
    - ***Version***: 1.2.1
    - ***App Size***: 6.1 MB
    - ***App Icon***:

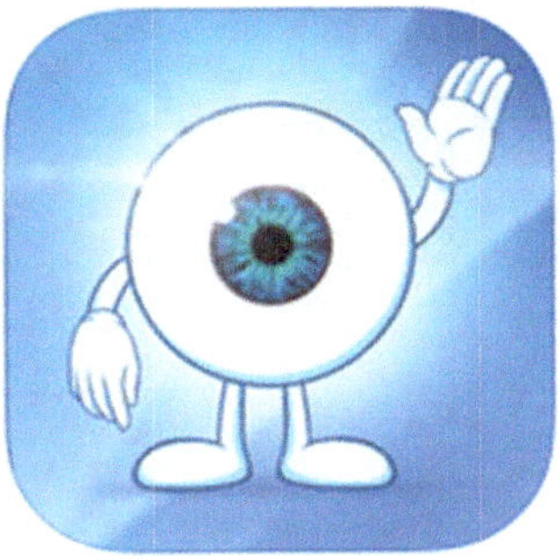

- ***App Screenshot***:

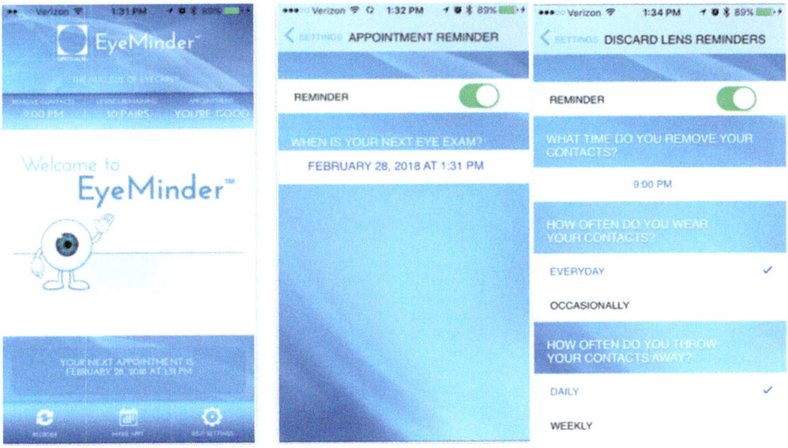

- ***Features***:
  This is also a reminder app which tells the user when to remove, replace and reorder their contact lenses.

QR Scanning Code for the App

iOS

Android

3. **Contact Lens Time**
   - ***Platform***: Android
   - ***App Creator***: Stefano Brandoli
   - ***Version***: 1.9.3
   - ***App Size***: 2.2 MB
   - ***App Icon***:

- *App Screenshots*:

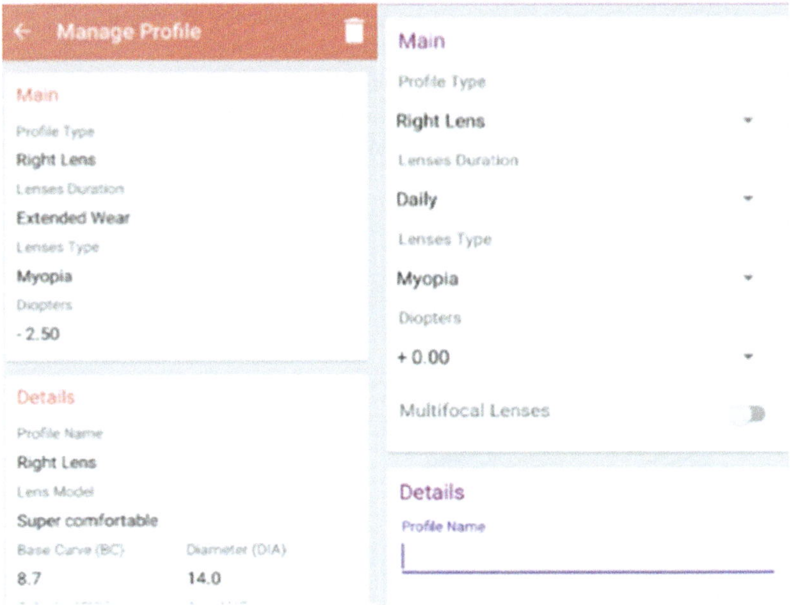

- ***Features***:
  This is similar to the previous app. The app is a contact lens manager that helps to remind the user when to change their contact lenses. It has the ability to separately manage the right and left eye. The app also provides information regarding contact lenses type, contact lenses duration, multifocal

  contact lenses model and colours, base curve, diameter, cylinder and axis for astigmatism.

  QR Scanning Code for the App

Or, if you have Siri, just tell her to remind you to change your contact lenses on X date every month, and she will let you know.

B. **Apps for Keratoconus**

Keratoconus is a degenerative corneal ectatic disorders characterized by progressive corneal thinning, protrusion and scarring. These eyes are characterized by higher-order aberrations due to the corneal changes, with numerous unusual, asymmetrical distortions. Just the sphere and cylinder components do not yield the best approximation to cancel out all the optical aberrations, and these patients need contact lenses over spectacles [1, 2]. Here are some mobile apps that may give reliable refraction.

1. **Helper Keratoconus**
   - ***Platforms***: iPhone; iPad
   - ***App Creator***: Evandro Souza
   - ***Version***: 2.0
   - ***App Size***: 3.7 MB
   - ***App Icon***:

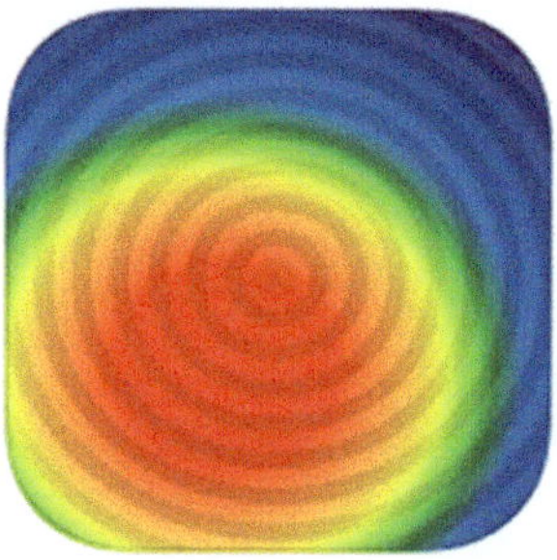

   - ***App Screenshot***:

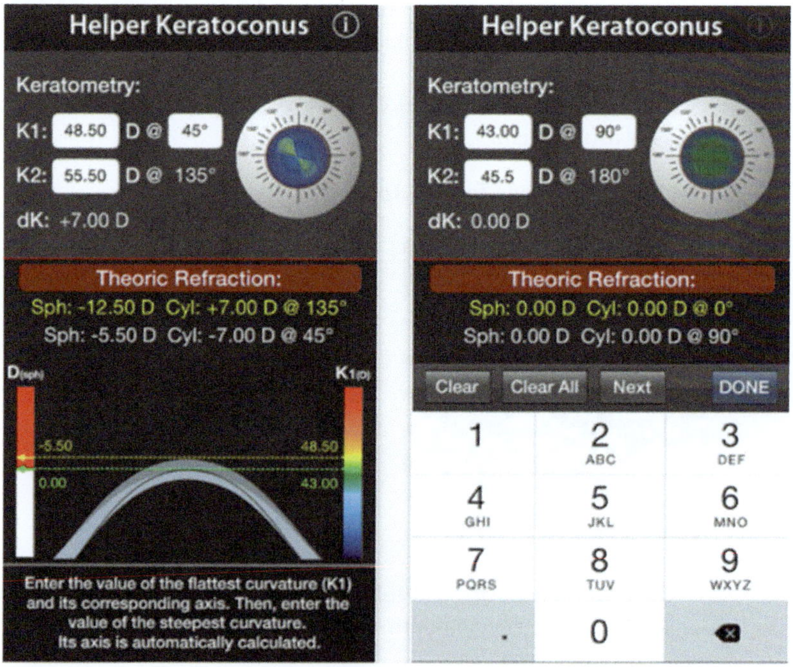

- ***Features***:
  Keratoconus hinders the reliable calculation of refraction of the patient due to the interference of higher-order aberrations generated by the irregular astigmatism.

  This app provides a theoretical calculation from patient keratometry refraction, which is fed into the refractor and refined.

  QR Scanning Code for the App

2. **Keratoconus Refraction Helper**
   - ***Platforms***: Android and iOS
   - ***App Creator***: Albertazzi Roberto
   - ***Version***: 1.0.0
   - ***App Size***: 11 Mb
   - ***App Icon***:

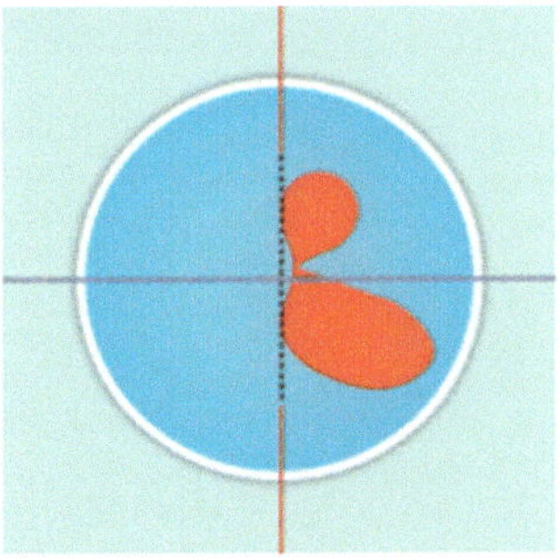

   - ***App Screenshots***:

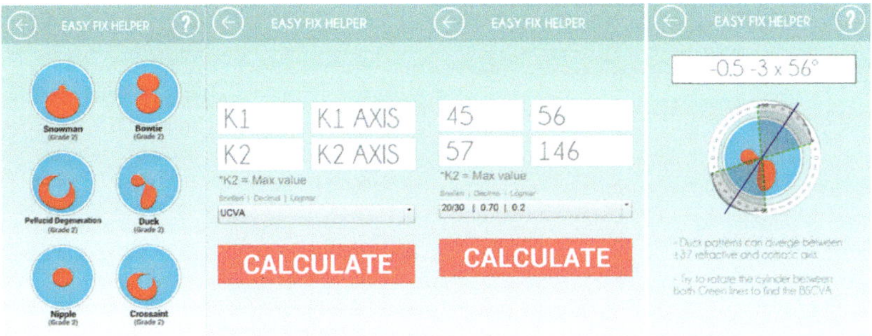

- ***Features***:
  This app is designed for axial length of 23 mm ± 0.5 mm, WTW (Wide-to-Wide) corneal diameter of 12 mm ± 1 mm and keratoconus grade 1 or 2 of Amsler-Krumeich classification. This app helps choose between the six different corneal topographies for the patient and based on that gives the best spectacle-corrected visual acuity, which is then used for the correction nomograms.

  QR Scanning Code for the App

  iOS Android

3. **Keratoconus Easy Fix**
   - ***Platforms***: Android
   - ***App Creator***: Albertazzi Roberto
   - ***Version***: 1.22
   - ***App Size***: 14 MB
   - ***App Icon***:

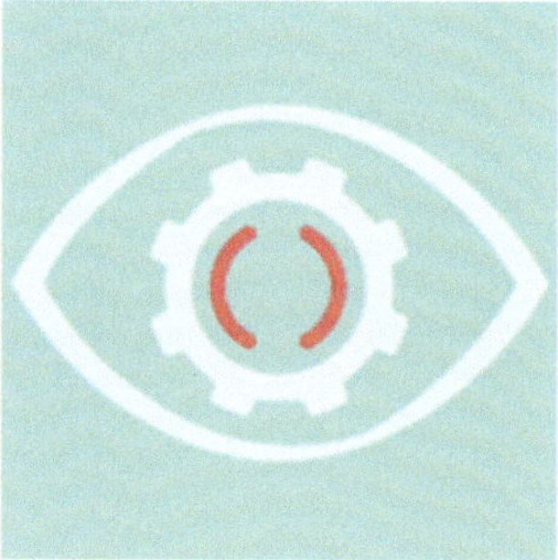

- ***App Screenshots***:

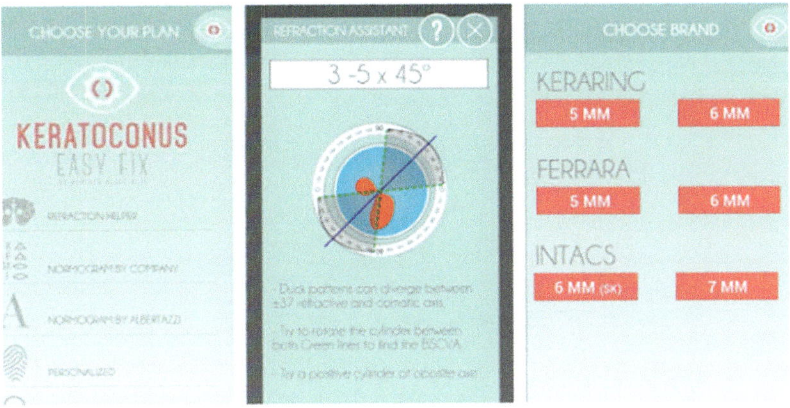

- ***Features***:
  This portable app is designed to aid in finding the proper intrastromal corneal ring segments (ICRS) for keratoconus surgery. It helps to check the intracorneal segment choices in the operating room or helps you choose the ICS to order for surgery. The app considers all nomograms.

  QR Scanning Code for the App

C. **Apps for Ocular Surface**
Dry eye is one of the most common ocular complaints with which people visit an ophthalmologist and is becoming increasingly prevalent with usage of desktop and handheld electronic devices. Many apps offer a tool, the Ocular Surface Disease Index (OSDI) questionnaire, that enables people to ascertain the severity of their dry eye condition by answering a series of simple questions about their ocular symptoms.

1. **OSDI**
   - ***Platforms***: Android (English, Spanish)
   - ***App Creator***: Yor
   - ***Version***:2.0

- ***App Size***: 1.6 MB
- ***App Icon***:

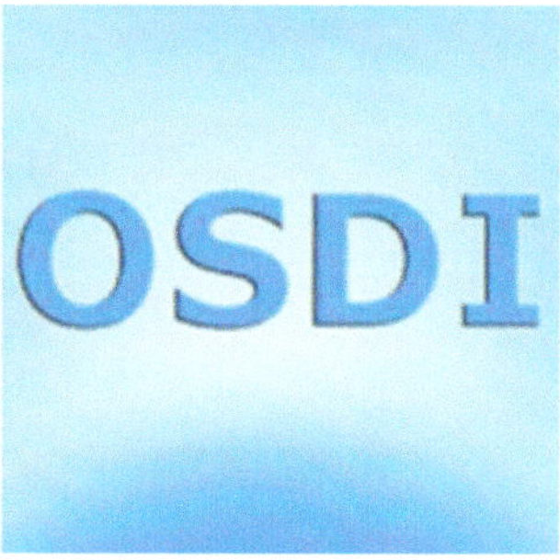

- ***App Screenshots***:

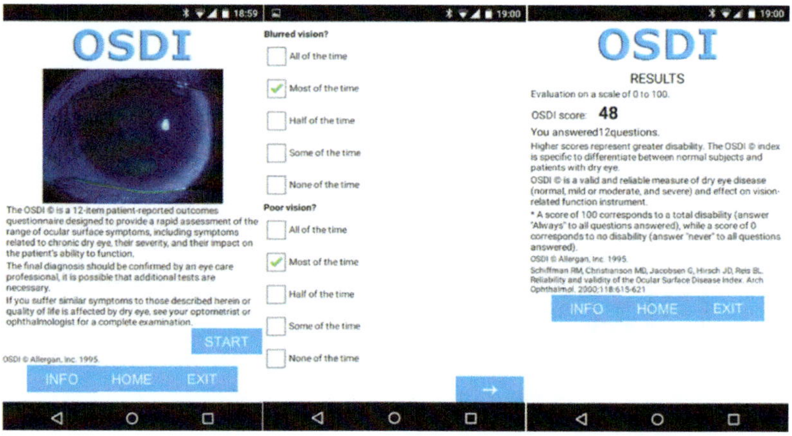

- ***Features***:

  The OSDI © is a 12-item patient-reported outcome questionnaire designed to provide a rapid assessment of the ocular surface symptoms, including symptoms related to chronic dry eye, their severity and their impact on the patient's ability to function.

  QR Scanning Code for the App

2. **Dry Eye OSDI Questionnaire**
   - ***Platforms***: iPhone
   - ***App Creator***: Allergan, Inc.
   - ***Version***: 1.0.3
   - ***App Size***: 12.7 MB
   - ***App Icon***:

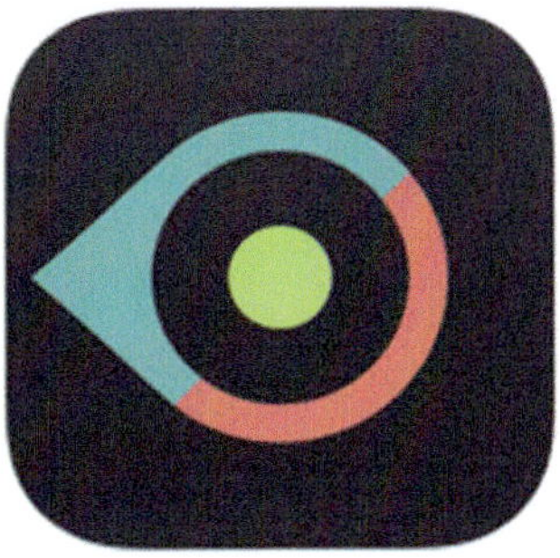

   - ***App Screenshot***:

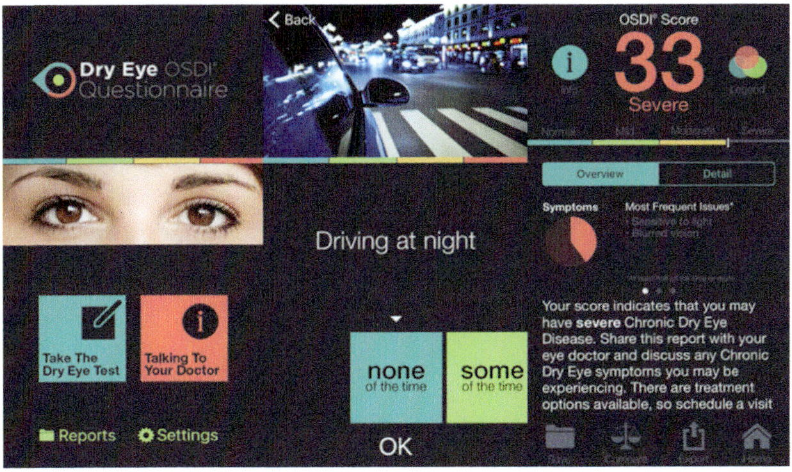

   - ***Features***:
     Similar to the previous app.

QR Scanning Code for the App

D. **Apps for Refractive Surgery**
   1. **LASIK**
      - ***Platforms***: Android
      - ***App Creator***: NABIOM SOFT
      - ***Version***: 1.0
      - ***App Size***: 27 MB
      - ***App Icon***:

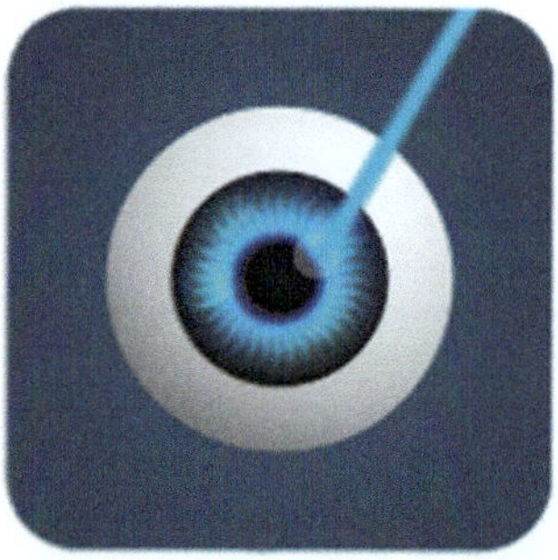

      - ***App Screenshots***:

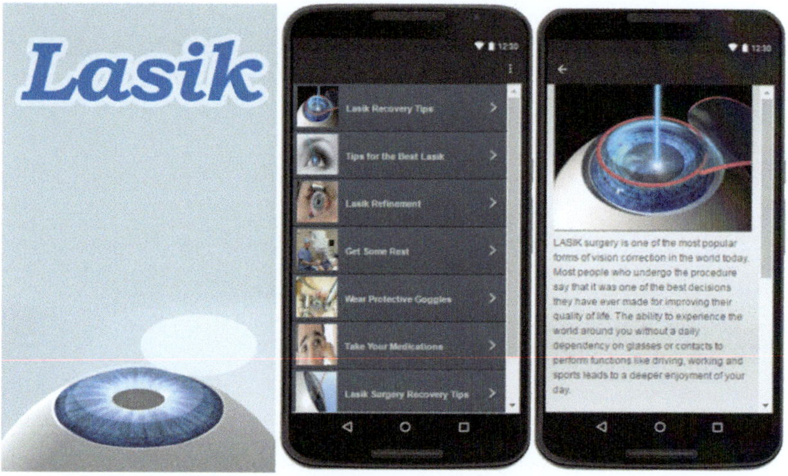

- ***Features***:
  This app is a one-stop shop for patients looking for basic information for refractive surgery, its advantages and disadvantages, opinions, outcome, etc.

  One must remember that this information is not a substitute for the one provided by your surgeon.

  QR Scanning Code for the App

2. **Lasik Safety Calculator**
   - ***Platforms***: Android
   - ***App Creator***: Jetbro
   - ***Version***: 1.0
   - ***App Size***: 1.1 MB
   - ***App Icon***:

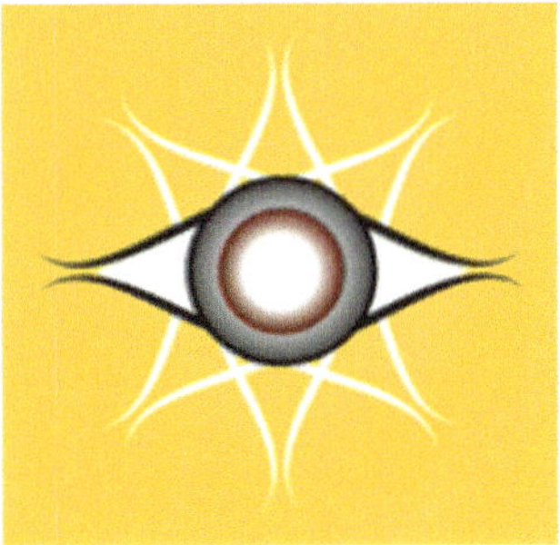

- ***App Screenshot***:

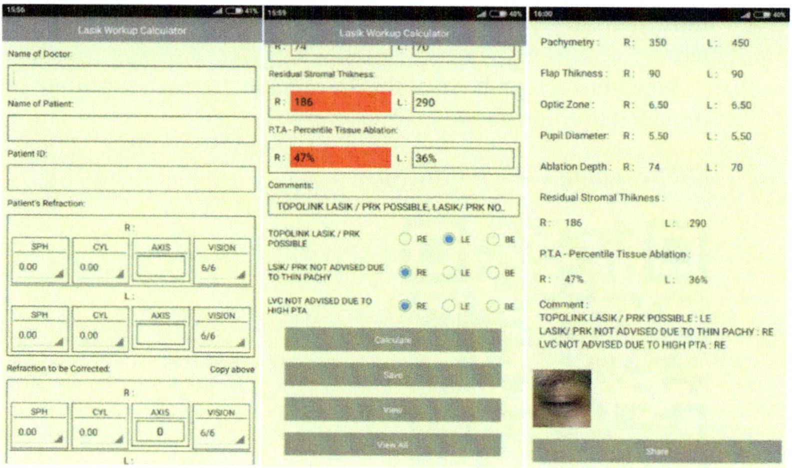

- ***Features***:
  This app was created to find out the possibility and safety of laser refractive surgery, namely, Smart Lasik, PRK and TopoLink Lasik. It is not meant for wavefront-guided customized Lasik. After entering patient's personal data, refraction of each eyes, keratectomy values, pachymetry of the cornea and type of refractive surgery, user can get RST (residual stromal thickness) and PTA (percentile of tissue ablated) and also get red highlighted field of keratectomy, RST and PTA if it is out of normal value. The user can also insert two images of each eye.

  QR Scanning Code for the App

3. **Moria Surgical**
   - ***Platforms***: Android
   - ***App Creator***: Veloce
   - ***Version***: 1.2.11.0
   - ***App Size***: 6.5 MB
   - ***App Icon***:

   - ***App Screenshots***:

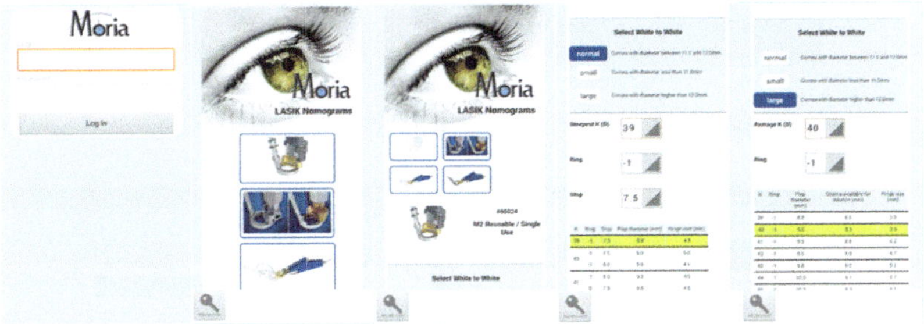

   - ***Features***:

     This app allows the ophthalmologist surgeons in the necessary calculations when using Moria LASIK equipment, Moria Nomograms. The surgeon can also send a request for a Moria-sponsored training session and for device warranty registration, using the app.

     QR Scanning Code for the App

4. **Pricelaser for LASIK Surgeons**
   - ***Platforms***: Android
   - ***App Creator***: Umbrella LLC
   - ***Version***: 1.0
   - ***App Size***: 0.96 MB
   - ***App Icon***:

   - ***App Screenshot***:

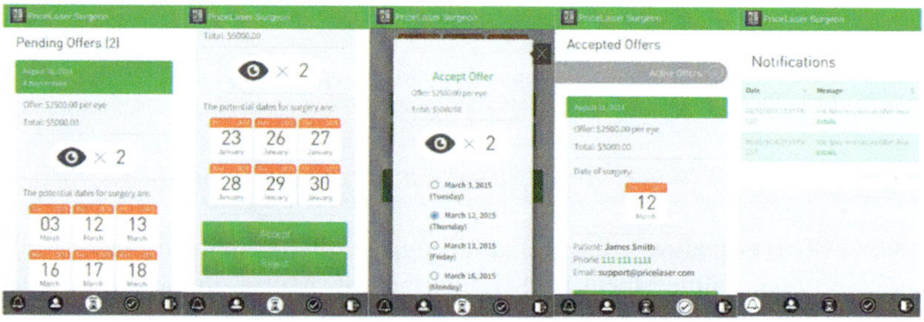

   - ***Features***:
     With this marketplace app prospective LASIK, PRK, LASEK and Epi-LASIK patients can connect with experienced, board-certified refractive eye surgeons at a price requested by the patient and accepted by the surgeon.

     QR Scanning Code for the App

Social Networking

A. ***Web Resources***

1. ***Cornea Society***

   The webpage of the Cornea Society keeps the anterior segment especially the corneal specialists updated through scientific meetings, communications and a quality scientific journal and newsletter.

   Website Screenshot

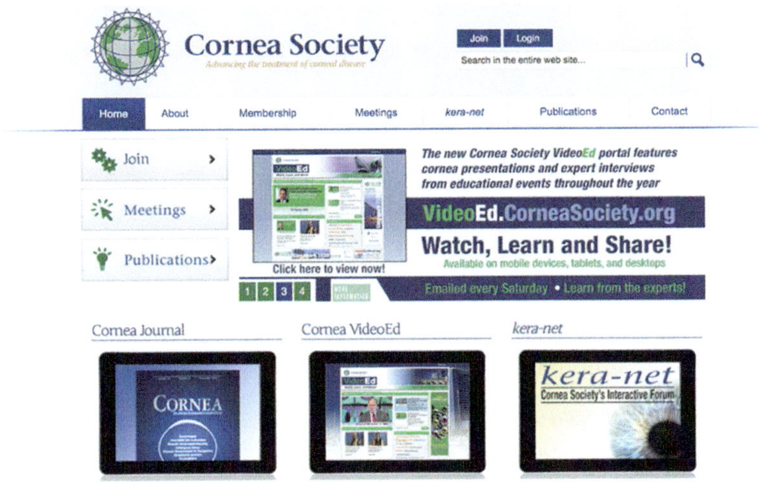

   ***Site URL**: http://www.corneasociety.org*

2. ***Cornea Society of India (CSI)***

   The CSI is an active society that formulates current practice patterns, facilitates fellowships and encourages scientific discussions with the goal to provide the best patient care and management.

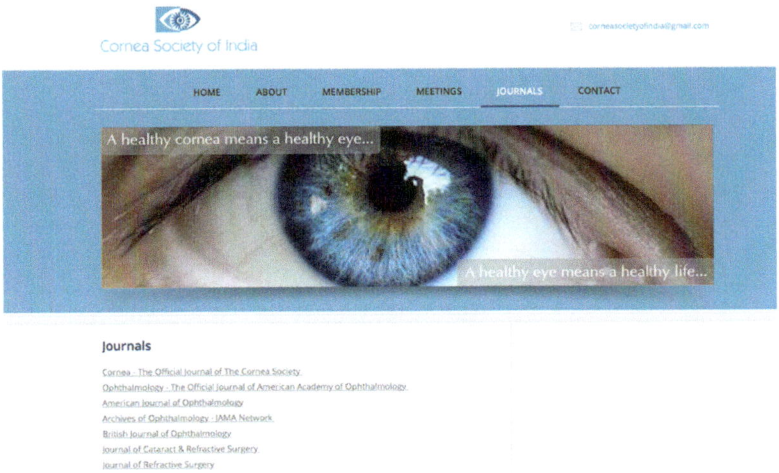

   ***Site URL**: http://www.corneasocietyindia.org*

3. ***British Society of Refractive Surgery***
   This webpage is a portal for British ophthalmologists, optometrists and others involved in all forms of refractive eye surgery. This group enables its members to exchange scientific information to keep abreast of developments.

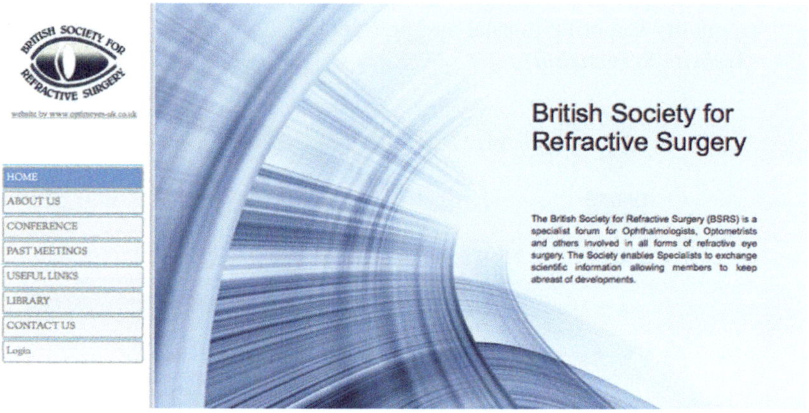

   ***Site URL**: http://www.bsrs.co.uk*

4. ***Cornea Research Foundation of America***
   It is a non-profit organization actively striving towards research and innovative treatment modalities for corneal disorders. Its Learning Centre and Medical Education section offers opportunities such as ALK Course, DMEK Course, PPV Course and much more for healthcare professionals.

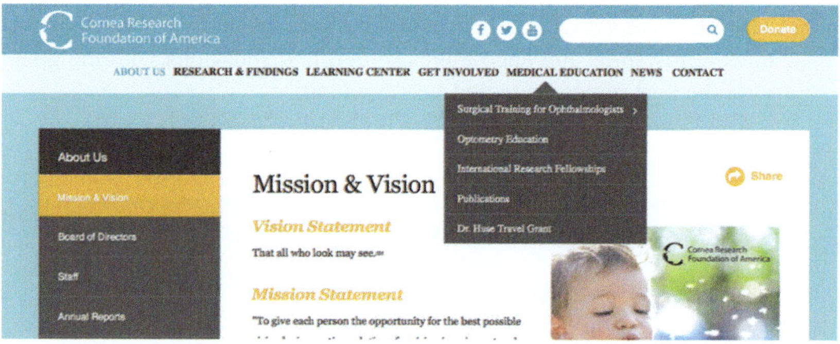

   ***Site URL**: http://www.cornea.org*

5. ***Eye Bank Association of America***
   Eye Bank Association of America is a non-profit organization that obtains, medically evaluates and distributes eyes donated for use in corneal transplantation, research and education. The webpage offers links for certification and recertification of Corneal Eye Bank Technicians and has a manual for guiding correct procedure for eye donation.
   Website Screenshot

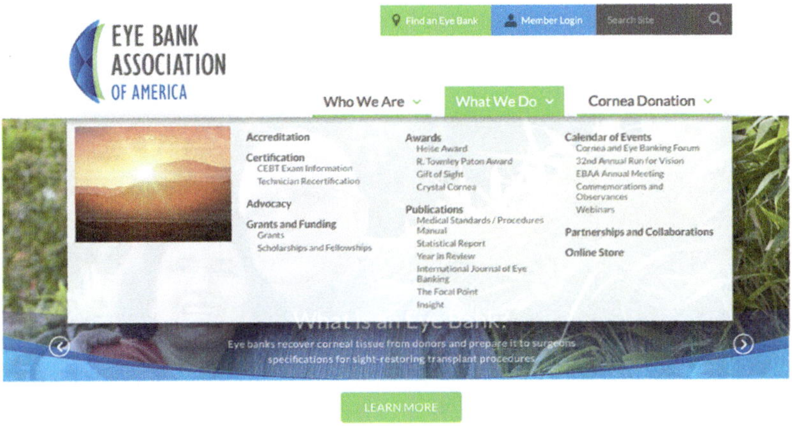

   Site URL**: **http://restoresight.org

6. ***Eye Bank Association of India (EBAI)***
   The official webpage of EBAI not only helps to increase awareness in eye donation and prevention of corneal blindness but also helps the ophthalmologists increase collection of eyes and introduce uniform standards in eye banks all over the country.
   Website Screenshot

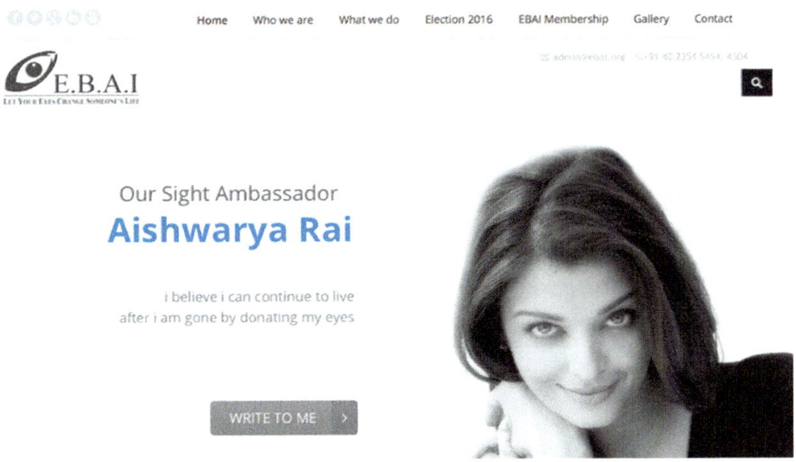

   Site URL**: **http://www.ebai.org

7. ***Millennial Eye***
   This is a webpage for the newer generation of tech savvy ophthalmologists. The webpage offers dynamic multimedia presentations and fully integrated social media. A wide array of topics ranging from practice management, career development, patient experience, industry collaboration and tech updates are addressed.
   Website Screenshot

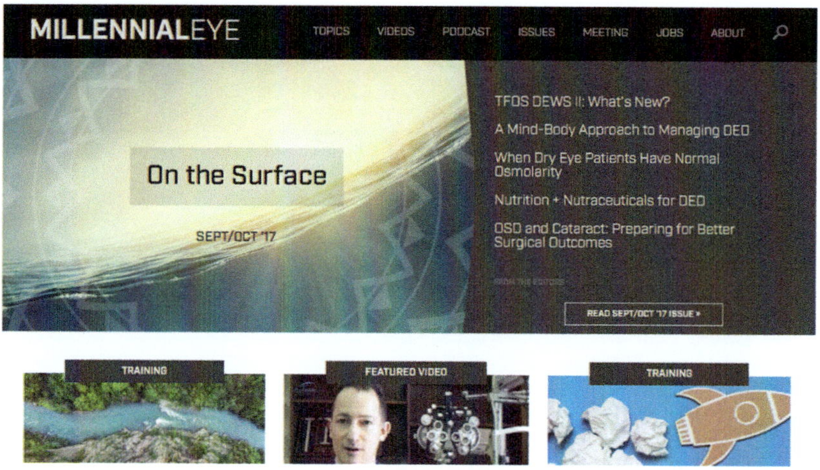

   Site URL**: **https://millennialeye.com

8. ***Eyetube***
   Eyetube is the largest online library of narrated, physician-created ophthalmic surgery videos on cataract, cornea, retina, glaucoma and refractive procedures and discussion from key opinion leaders.
   Website Screenshot

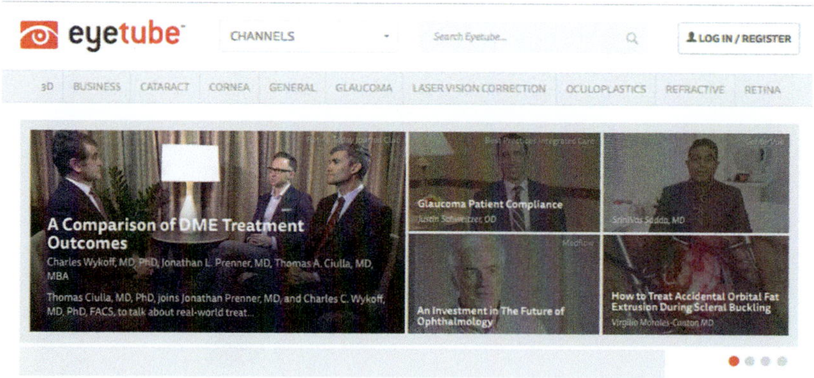

   Site URL**: **https://eyetube.net

B. *Facebook Pages*

S. No	Page icon	Page name	Description	QR code
Society pages				
1.		EuCornea—European Society of Cornea and Ocular Surface Disease Specialists	Promotes the dissemination of the highest level of knowledge in the field of cornea and ocular surface disease among ophthalmologists and the public	
2.		Indian Society of Cornea and Keratore-fractive Surgeons—ISCKRS	Posts updates regarding the society's meetings	
3.		Keratoconus society	Provides up-to-date information on treatment options for keratoconus, both for profes-sionals and patients	
4.		National Keratoconus Foundation	This page increases awareness for treatment of keratoconus for individuals diagnosed with keratoconus and their families	

(continued)

S. No	Page icon	Page name	Description	QR code
Patient support groups				
1.		Corneal Transplant Foundation @cornealtrans-plantfoundation	Official FB page of a non-profit organization that assists economically disadvantaged patients in obtaining corneal transplants, supports research related to corneal transplant procedures and material and provides information about corneal transplant procedures	
2.		Keratomania-Keratoconus Support and Awareness	Raises awareness about keratoconus and other corneal ectatic disorders	
3.		Keratoconus Group @Keratoconus-group	The largest keratoconus community, for patients and specialists	
4.	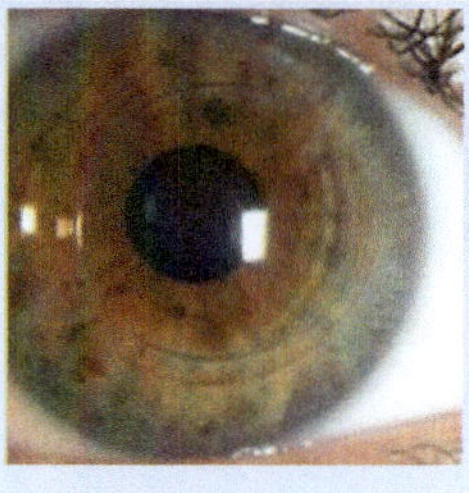	INTACS(ICRS) Keratoconus Treatment @Keratoconus treatment-INTACS	Shares the techniques and updates about INTACS	

S. No	Page icon	Page name	Description	QR code
5.		Corneal Dystrophy Foundation	Through this page this foundation shares educational information and webinars. They also regularly schedule symposium with experts in the field of corneal dystrophies	

C. *Twitter Handles*

S. No	Handle icon	Handle name	Description	QR code
1.		SightLife Surgical @SLSurgical	Handle for a non-profit global health organization solely focused on eliminating corneal blindness worldwide	
2.		Keratoconus GB @KeratoconusGB	News and chat for patients with keratoconus	
3.		Dry Eye Coach	This handle is an ocular surface information hub	

S. No	Handle icon	Handle name	Description	QR code
4.	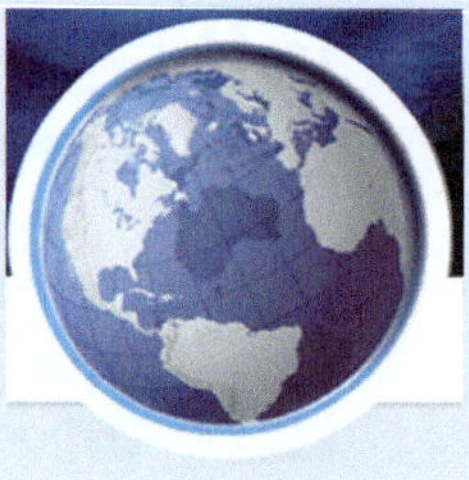	Eye World @EWNews	Links for ongoing innovations in surgical procedures and practice trends	

It is increasingly becoming evident how smartphone applications and web resources are aiding ophthalmologists. As the technology continues to evolve, the number of apps focussed for each subspeciality will only increase.

References

1. Gore DM, Shortt AJ, Allan BD. New clinical pathways for Keratoconus. Eye. 2013;27:329–39.
2. Andreanos KD, Hashemi K, Petrelli M, Droutsas K, Georgalas I, Kymionis GD. Keratoconus treatment algorithm. Ophthalmol Ther. 2017;6(2):245–62.

Apps and Social Networking Pages for Strabismus and Paediatric Ophthalmology

7

Paediatric ophthalmology is one of the most important subspecialities that cater to children's eye health. This is an important and challenging issue across the world. The World Health Organization (WHO) has identified childhood blindness and genetic eye diseases as priority eye diseases as a part of its global eye health action plan for 2014–2019. It is challenging to treat paediatric eye diseases as vision impairment may result from the disease entity per se, or from disruption of the normal visual and neurological developmental processes, or a combination of both.

Screening and early intervention is required to minimize the impact of the eye disorder on the developing visual system. If left untreated, this visual impairment continues into adulthood and working life, causing substantial impact on the child's quality of life. Children with chronic paediatric eye diseases like congenital/developmental glaucoma have quality-of-life scores similar to those seen in children with severe congenital cardiac anomalies, who have undergone liver transplants or who have acute lymphoblastic leukaemia [1].

In this chapter we discuss the use of mobile technology for screening, diagnosis and treatment of paediatric eye diseases. The app approach to paediatric eye care can definitely make the ophthalmologist's job a lot easier while making it fun and engaging for this very demanding patient subset.

Applications

The apps will be discussed under the following heads:

A. Physician resources
B. Amblyopia management
C. App for convergence insufficiency

P. Ichhpujani, S. Thakur, *Smart Resources in Ophthalmology*, Current Practices in Ophthalmology, https://doi.org/10.1007/978-981-13-0140-7_7

A. **Physician Resources**

1. ***AAPOS Vision Screening App ($29.99)***
   - ***Platforms***: iOS (iPad only)
   - ***App Creator***: Good-Lite Company
   - ***Version***: 1.1
   - ***App Size***: 5 MB
   - ***App Icon***:

   - ***App Screenshots***:

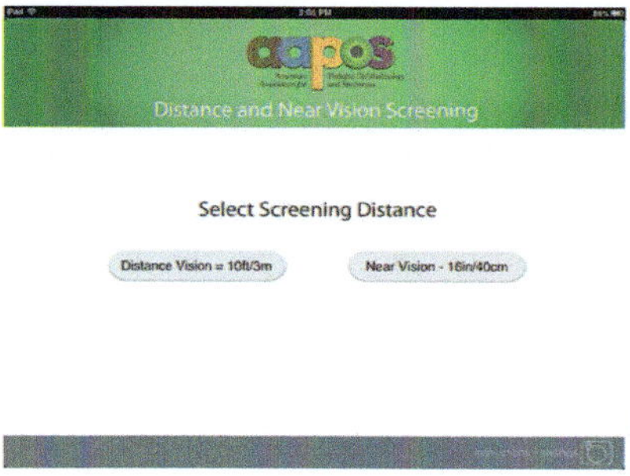

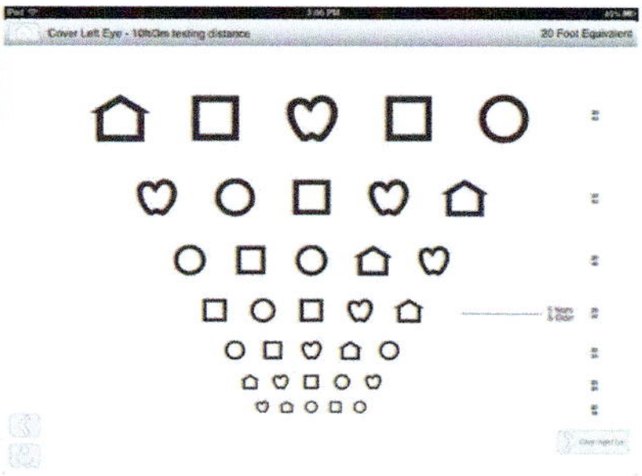

   - ***Features***:

The app is based on the basic distance Vision Screening Kit, created by the American Association of Pediatric Ophthalmology and Strabismus (AAPOS). Charts include both full-chart threshold and critical line formats using either Sloan Letters optotypes or LEA Symbols. Critical line screening is a quick method for screening where individuals are screened using only the line that matches their age. Each test format can be used for distance screening at 10 ft/3 m or for near vision screening at 16 in./40 cm. Each screening test starts with a practice screen to familiarize the user with the process, followed by the screening test for first the right eye and then the left eye. The pass/fail criterion is indicated for the age group in each screen.

QR Scanning Codes for the App

2. ***JPOS***
   - ***Platforms***: iOS
   - ***App Creator***: The Wyanoke Group
   - ***Version***: 1.0
   - ***App Size***: 44 MB
   - ***App Icon***:

- ***App Screenshots***:

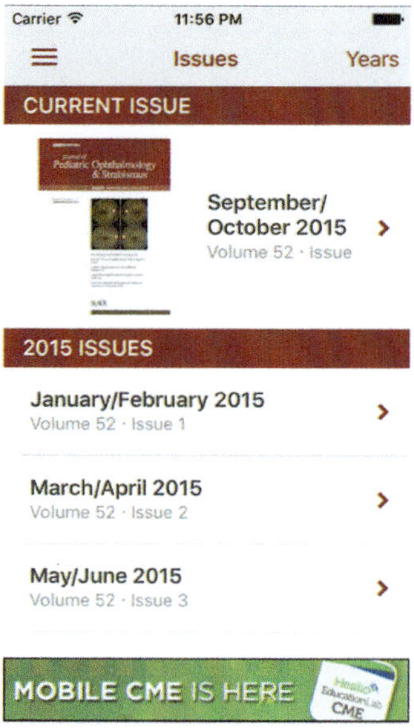

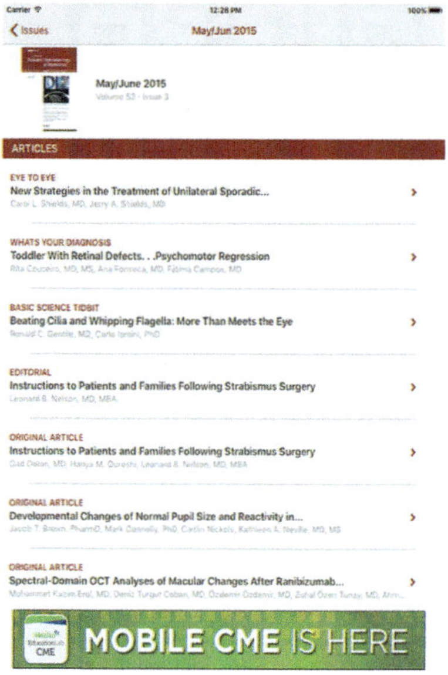

- ***Features***:
  This application offers the mobile reader an experience of the *Journal of Pediatric Ophthalmology and Strabismus*. This bimonthly peer-reviewed journal publishes original articles on the diagnosis, treatment and prevention of eye disorders in the paediatric age group and the treatment of strabismus in all age groups. The JPOS app has features like Eye to Eye, What's Your Diagnosis?, Basic Science Titbit and Images in Pediatric Ophthalmology. The application is free trial based, but continued usage requires in-application purchase of the journal subscription.

  QR Scanning Code for the App

3. ***Strabismus Surgery ($11.99)***
   - ***Platforms***: iOS and Android
   - ***App Creator***: MedHand Mobile Libraries
   - ***Version***: 2.3.1
   - ***App Size***: 11.8 MB
   - ***App Icon***:

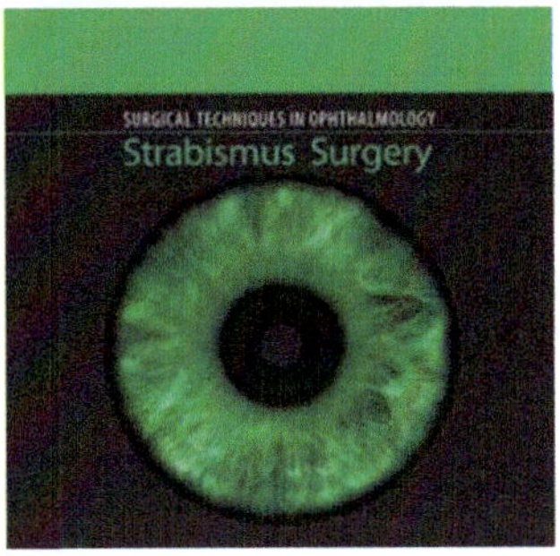

   - ***App Screenshots***:

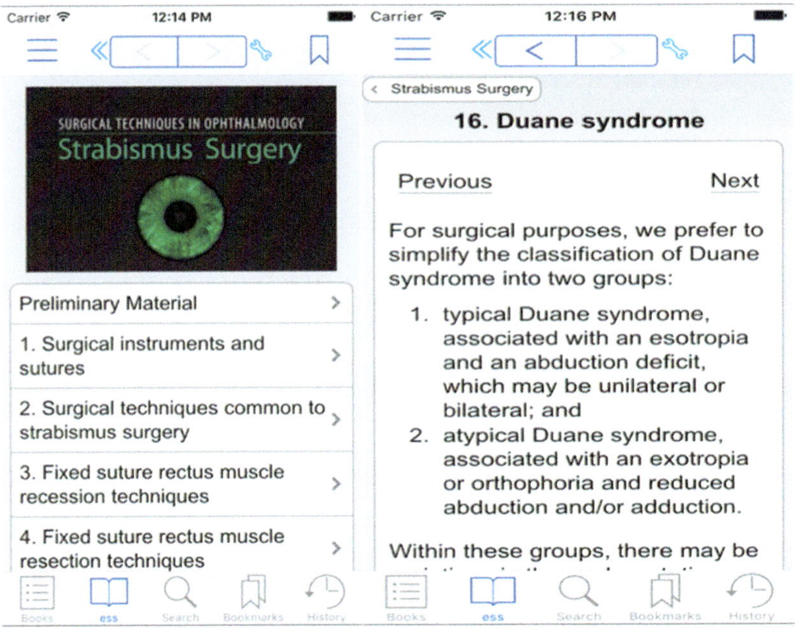

   - ***Features***:
     This is a mobile-optimized version of the textbook, *Surgical Techniques in Ophthalmology Series*, authored by John D. Ferris and Peter E. J. Davies. It features the essential information you need on a variety of surgical

manoeuvres in paediatric ophthalmology. Authoritative, exhaustive and easily digestible, this is one application that every POS resident needs to be on the top. The illustrations are both line art and clinical images which make this application a visual treat.

QR Scanning Code for the App

iOS Android

4. ***StrabisPIX***
   - ***Platforms***: Android
   - ***App Creator***: Boston Children's Hospital
   - ***Version***: 2.3.1
   - ***App Size***: 11.8 MB
   - ***App Icon***:

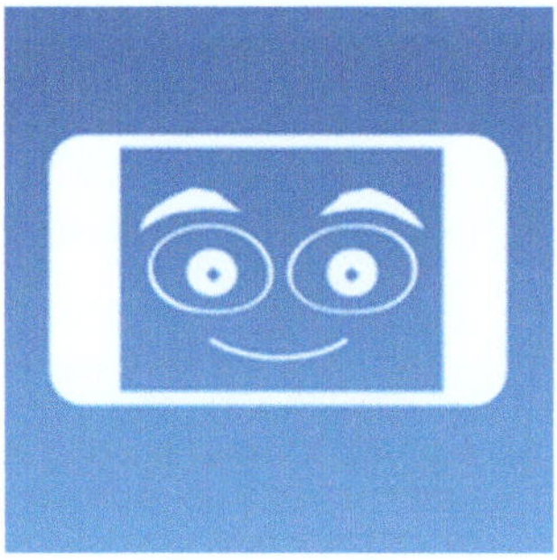

- ***App Screenshots***:

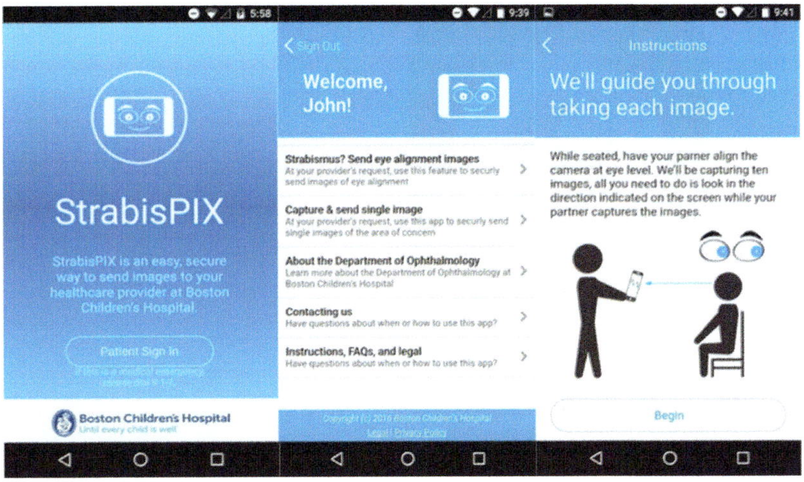

- ***Features***:
  This is an easy, secure way to send images of eye gaze or areas of concern to Boston Children's Hospital. The application is an excellent way of data collection that can be adopted worldwide. With the advent of excellent imaging capabilities, teleophthalmology for squint referral is not a distant dream anymore.
  QR Scanning Code for the App

5. ***Smart Optometry (Free with Ads and In-App Purchases)***
   - ***Platforms***: Android and iOS
   - ***App Creator***: Smart Optometry
   - ***Version***: 3.5
   - ***App Size***: 114 MB

- ***App Icon***:

- ***App Screenshots***:

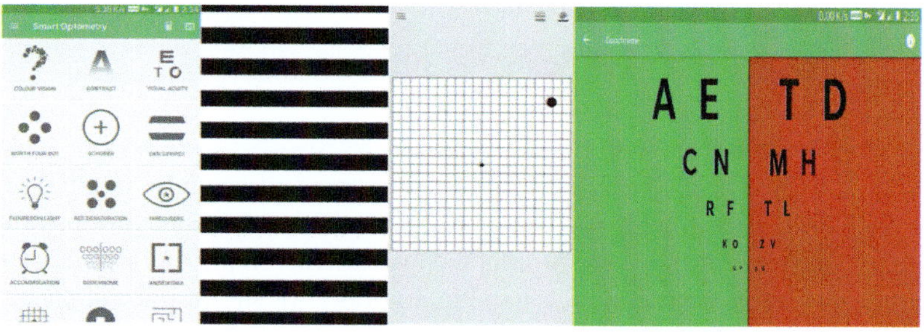

- ***Features***:
  This is a free application with in-app ads, which can be used to assess the colour vision, contrast, visual acuity, Worth four dot test, Schober test, OKN stripes, red desaturation test and the Hirschberg test. In addition to these, the app can assess accommodation and aniseikonia and also has an Amsler grid. The application is available in English, Spanish, German, French, Italian, Polish, Norwegian, Croatian, Slovenian, Czech and Russian. The application has a simple user interface and all the tests are interactive.

  QR Scanning Code for the App

iOS

Android

6. ***StereoAcuity Test—Cardboard***
   - ***Platforms***: Android
   - ***App Creator***: cs.unibg
   - ***Version***: 1.0.9
   - ***App Size***: 1.21 MB
   - ***App Icon***:

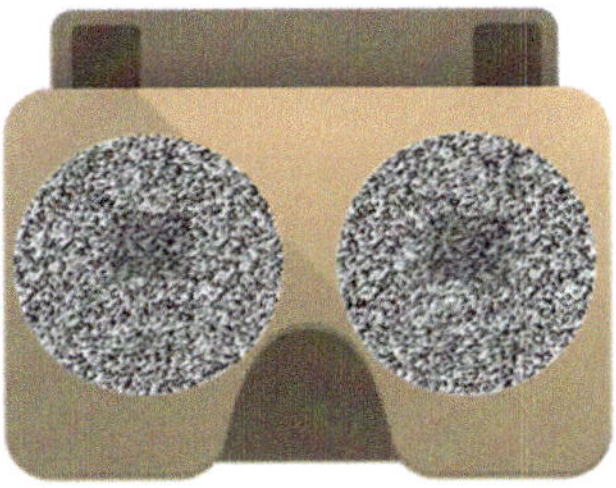

   - ***App Screenshots***:

   - ***Features***:
     This is a free VR-based application. It is based on the Randot stereoacuity test. The left eye sees one set of dots and the right eye sees a second set of dots. The dots are identical except for the dots within the shape that have been horizontally displaced. Amblyopic people may not be able to recognize the images, and thus the application can be used to screen a population for people with amblyopia. The image shows a child undergoing the test using a VR device.

     QR Scanning Code for the App

7. ***9Gaze***
   - ***Platforms***: iOS
   - ***App Creator***: SeeVision LLC
   - ***Version***: 1.0
   - ***App Size***: 27.5 MB
   - ***App Icon***:

   - ***App Screenshots***:

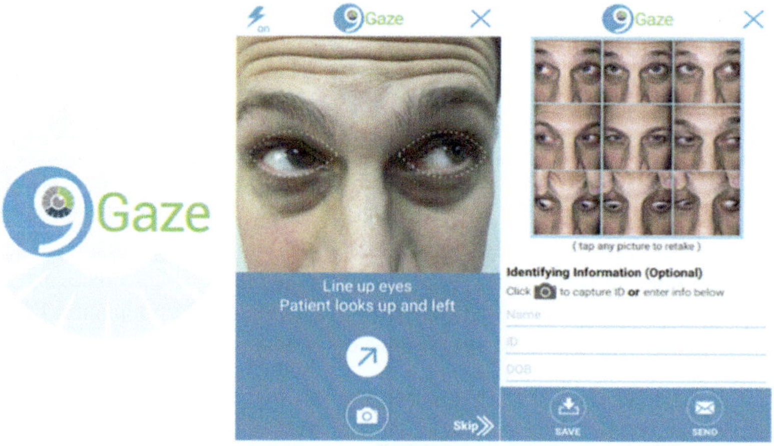

   - ***Features***:
     This is an easy, quick and efficient way to document eye motility and strabismus in the nine cardinal positions of gaze. The app provides an on-screen guide for eye positioning to assist with image consistency through all nine photographs. 9Gaze app automatically creates a composite image of the nine photographs for easy exporting. One can email the image to oneself for importing into electronic medical record or save to camera roll.

QR Scanning Code for the App

8. ***eyeTilt***
   - ***Platforms***: iOS
   - ***App Creator***: SeeVision LLC
   - ***Version***: 1.0
   - ***App Size***: 16.5 MB
   - ***App Icon***:

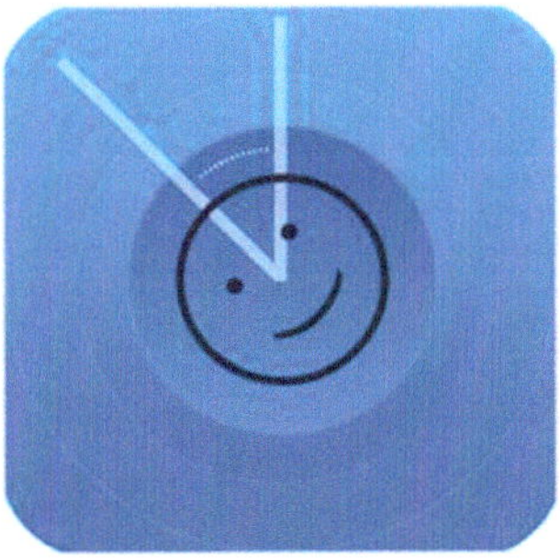

   - ***App Screenshots***:

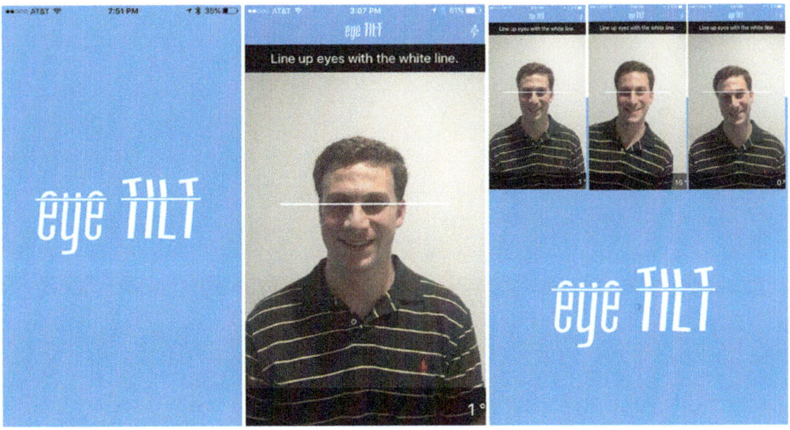

- ***Features***:
  This is an easy, quick and efficient app to determine how many degrees someone's head is tilted. Before eyeTilt, physicians used a goniometer to estimate the degree of head turn. Now, you can use your iPhone or iPad to measure head tilt. Just hold up your device, line up the eyes, and the device will tell you the tilt of the head. Use for strabismus, torticollis or any other way you would like.

  QR Scanning Code for the App

9. ***Park Three Step (1.99$)***
   - ***Platforms***: iOS
   - ***App Creator***: Todd Zarwell
   - ***Version***: 1.01
   - ***App Size***: 4.8 MB
   - ***App Icon***:

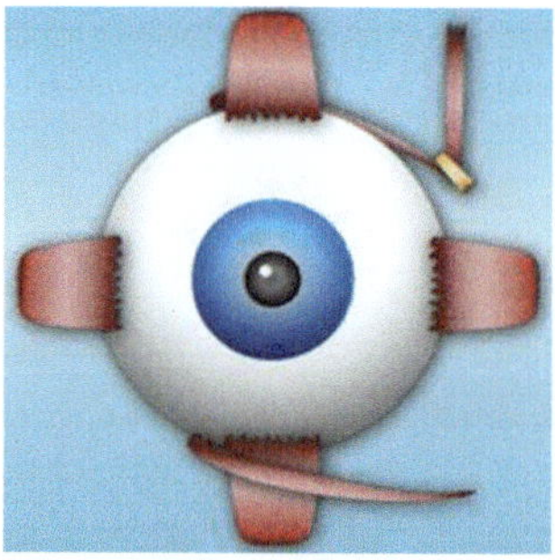

- ***App Screenshots***:

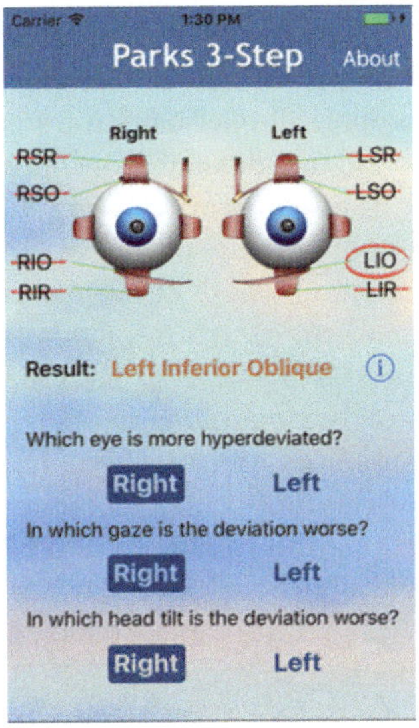

- ***Features***:
  Park's three-step test is used to isolate the paretic muscle in acquired vertical diplopia. When the doctor enters his/her observations for each of the three tests, then the app suggests which extraocular muscle is underacting.

  QR Scanning Code for the App

B. **Amblyopia Management**

Amblyopia has been the still unconquered realm in ophthalmology for quite a long time. Requiring dedicated follow-up and unprecedented cooperation from patients and caregivers, every paediatric ophthalmologist fears this condition the most. Despite the availability of meticulous surgical intervention for paediatric eye diseases, it is often the postoperative period that defines surgical outcome.

With renewed interest and excellent results reported from literature, dichoptic training and perceptual learning are being explored as a modality for amblyopia management, especially in adults where conventional patching is often unsuccessful [2–5]. The mechanism of action of this treatment modality is uncertain, but video games have been shown to induce neuronal plasticity that can aid in reprograming of the neural networks [6]. This reprograming can hence help in restoration of vision in amblyopic patients. Binocular video gameplay as a modality of amblyopia management has been compared to patching and has shown encouraging results [7, 8]. While you can find several applications on the Google Play Store or the iOS store that mimic the dichoptic training games that aid in amblyopia management, we here shall limit our discussion to those which have been clinically validated and are free to use.

1. ***Duovision***
   - ***Platforms***: iOS and Android
   - ***App Creator***: Melios
   - ***Version***: 1.1.6
   - ***App Size***: 5 MB
   - ***App Icon***:

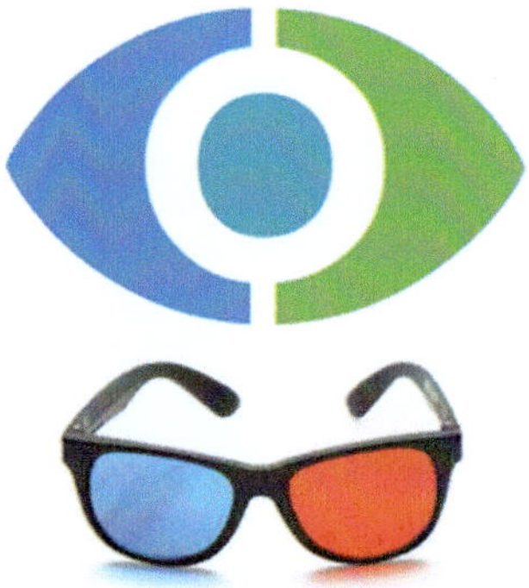

- ***App Screenshots***:

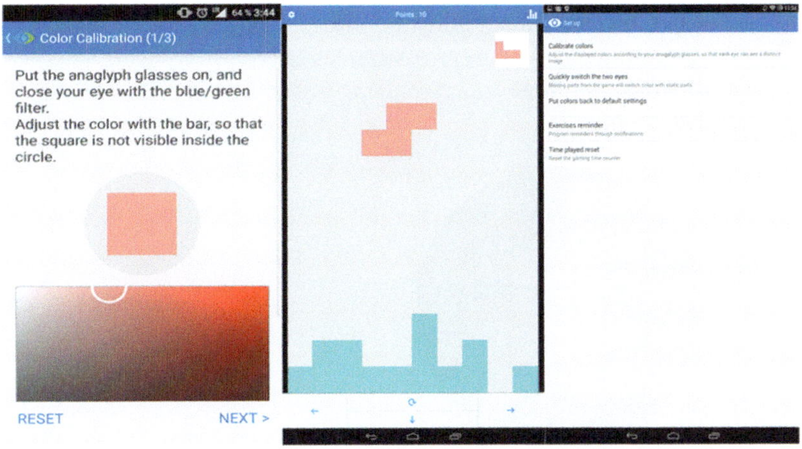

- ***Features***:

The app is based on the fact that each eye sees a different image and the amblyopic eye works in coordination with the 'valid' eye, playing a video game. To play, each eye must send information to the brain, and this forces the amblyopic eye to work. The app requires anaglyph glasses that are then used to selectively present objects to either eye. In a multicentre, randomized clinical trial on 385 children (aged 5–13 years) with amblyopia (20/40 to 20/200) strabismic, anisometropic or both, a similar application was used. At 16 weeks, mean amblyopic eye VA improved 1.05 lines in the game group and 1.35 lines in the patching group, with an adjusted treatment group difference of 0.31 lines favouring patching, though only 39 of the 176 participants (22.2%) randomized to the binocular game performed more than 75% of the prescribed treatment [8].

The results are promising and encourage more studies that use graphically engaging games, which can improve compliance and effectiveness of video game-based treatment for amblyopia [7].

QR Scanning Codes for the App

iOS Android

2. ***Amblyopia Games***
   - ***Platforms***: Android
   - ***App Creator***: Minian Software Ltd
   - ***Version***: 1.0
   - ***App Size***: 44 MB
   - ***App Icon***:

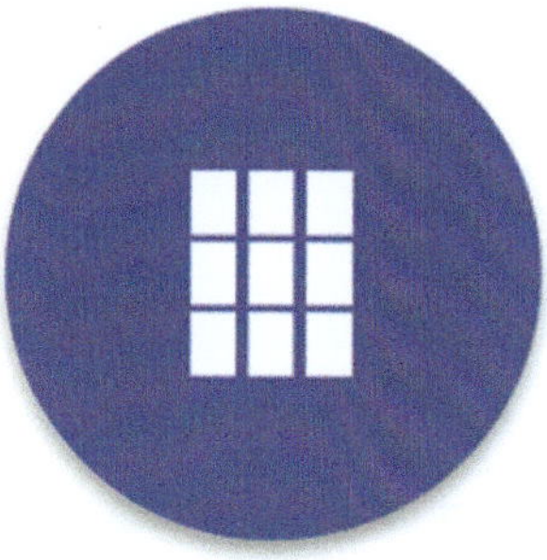

   - ***App Screenshots***:

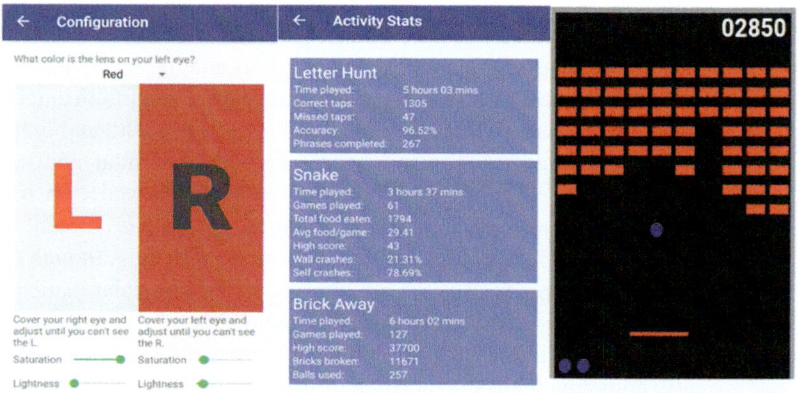

   - ***Features***:
     This application offers several inbuilt games that are based on the principle of dichoptic training. Games like Brick Breaker, Snake and Tetris make sure that there's always something new to improve the patient compliance. The ability to control the saturation and contrast of the colours gives additional control over the degree of treatment offered.

QR Scanning Code for the App

3. ***Car Race Cardboard***
    - ***Platforms***: Android
    - ***App Creator***: ca.unibg
    - ***Version***: 1.1
    - ***App Size***: 9.75 MB
    - ***App Icon***:

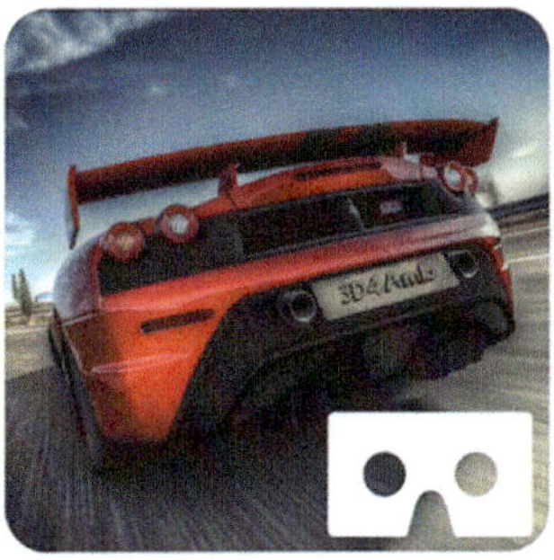

- ***App Screenshots***:

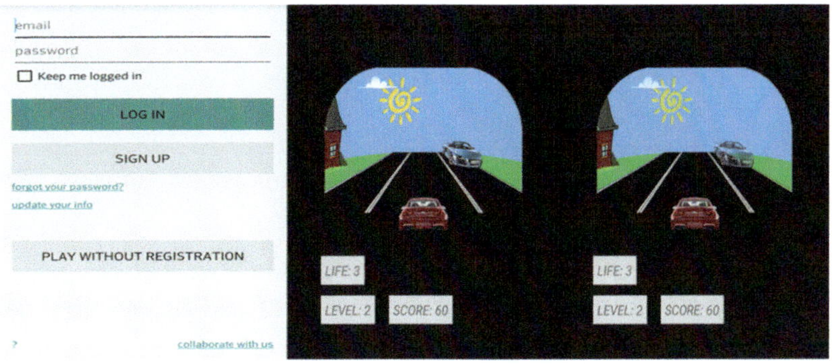

- ***Features***:
  This application uses a VR headset to give an immersive experience to the user. More immersion should translate into better compliance. This application offers a very basic proof of this concept [9]. Though very expensive devices like the Vivid Vision platform offer better graphics, this application is an encouraging sign of times to come [10]. The developers of this application are very active and can be contacted for collaboration via the QR code given below.

  QR Scanning Code for the App

  Game

  Developer Website

C. **App for Convergence Insufficiency**
   1. ***MyEyeGym***
      - ***Platforms***: Android
      - ***App Creator***: Singapore National Eye Centre
      - ***Version***: 1.4.2
      - ***App Size***: 38.7 MB
      - ***App Icon***:

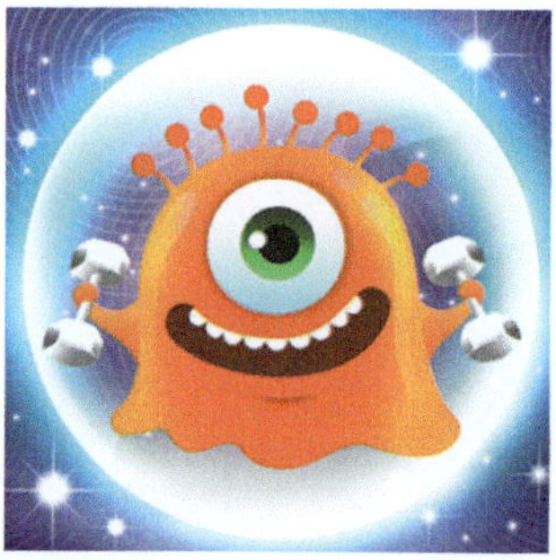

- ***App Screenshots***:

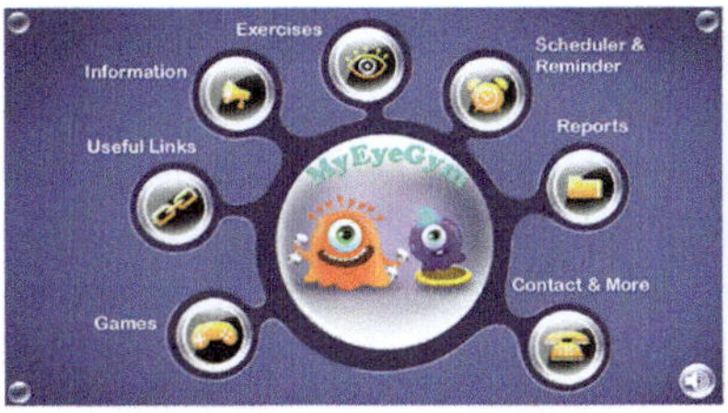

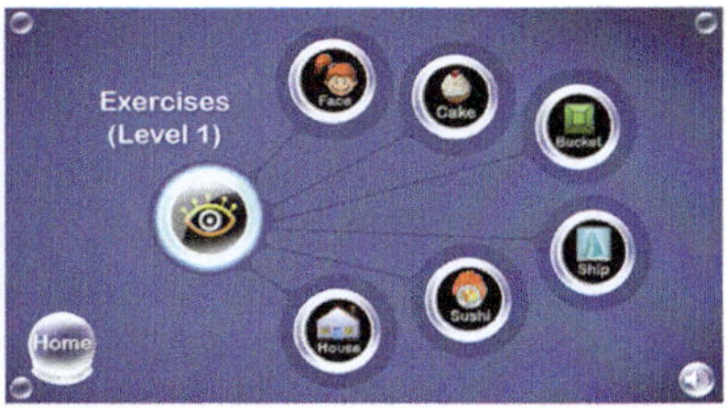

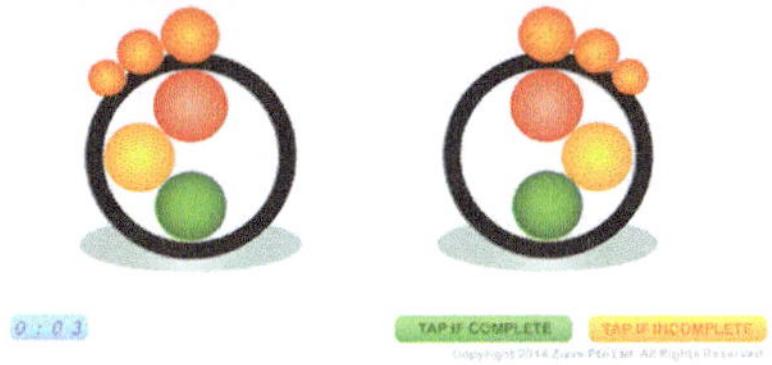

- ***Features***:
MyEyeGym is an orthoptic eye exercise app for people who have an intermittent squint with difficulty maintaining good eye alignment. MyEyeGym is suitable for horizontal, non-paretic and intermittent types of strabismus. Research has shown that performing fusion exercise is effective in improving the binocular status of people with certain types of strabismus [11, 12]. This application uses stereogram images to exercise the eye muscles. Additionally it has tools for tracking and recording compliance like notifications and alerts.

QR Scanning Codes for the App

Social Networking

A. ***Web Resources***

1. ***AAPOS***: AAPOS is the American Association for Pediatric Ophthalmology and Strabismus. The organization's goals are to advance the quality of children's eye care, support the training of paediatric ophthalmologists, support research activities in paediatric ophthalmology and advance the care of adults with strabismus. The website offers a lot of resources like presentations and vision screening kits for healthcare providers. Additionally, the website has a patient knowledge data pool that is regularly updated.
Website Screenshots

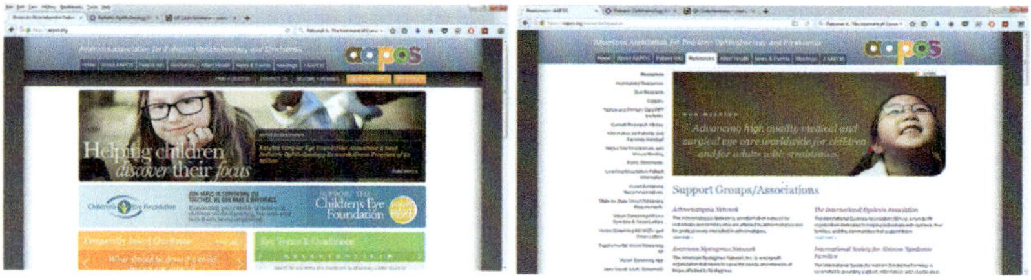

Site URL: https://aapos.org

2. ***AAO Paediatric Ophthalmology: One Network***: This webpage offers the best content on paediatric ophthalmology; however the multimedia content requires an AAO subscription. This is one of the best places to get the latest information about the subspeciality.
Website Screenshots

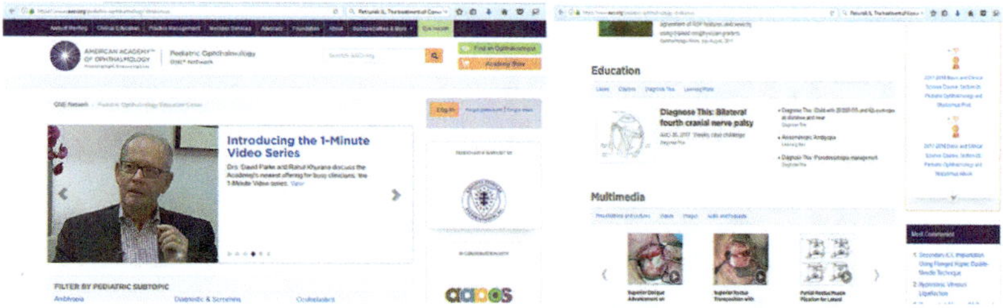

Site URL: https://www.aao.org/pediatric-ophthalmology-strabismus

3. ***International Strabismological Association***: The International Strabismological Association (ISA) was formed in 1966. ISA holds scientific meeting every 4 years in a different part of the world. The website offers a sneak peek into the history of strabismology and has a lot of resources on strabismus diagnosis and management.

Website Screenshots

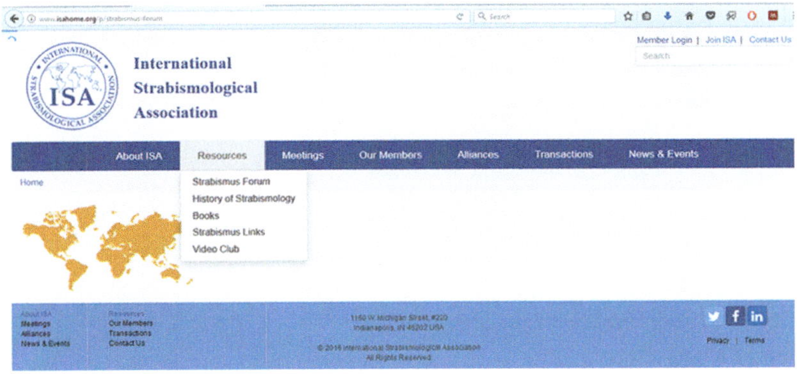

Site URL: http://www.isahome.org/

4. ***World Society of Paediatric Ophthalmology and Squint***: The World Society of Paediatric Ophthalmology and Strabismus (WSPOS) is a registered charity. Any individual interested or involved in paediatric ophthalmology and strabismus care can become a member for free. The WSPOS has introduced a concept of connectivity based on the development of a network of like-minded individuals or groups, driven by goals of education, training and research. The website has podcasts, surgical videos, paper abstracts and other educational resources for those engaged in paediatric ophthalmology.

Website Screenshots

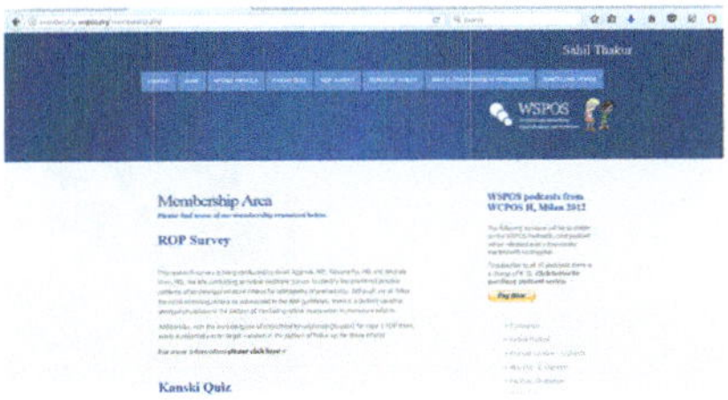

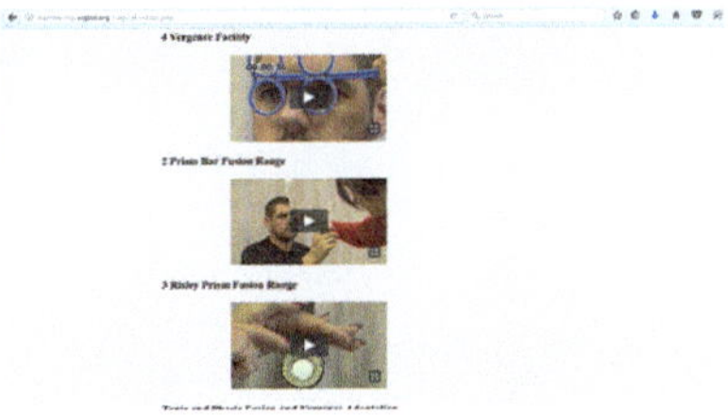

Site URL: http://wspos.org

5. ***Cybersight***: Cybersight is a not-for-profit telemedicine initiative founded by Orbis International to help mitigate the shortage of skilled eye health professionals in developing countries and help those in remote areas combat geographic isolation. With advanced online training tools and access to international expert faculty and trainers, Cybersight continues to connect professionals, clinics, hospitals, health systems and NGOs to reduce the global burden of avoidable blindness. It has excellent resources on paediatric ophthalmology and is free to use. The website offers classic texts in pdf format, and credits for the courses can be printed as transcripts.

Website Screenshots

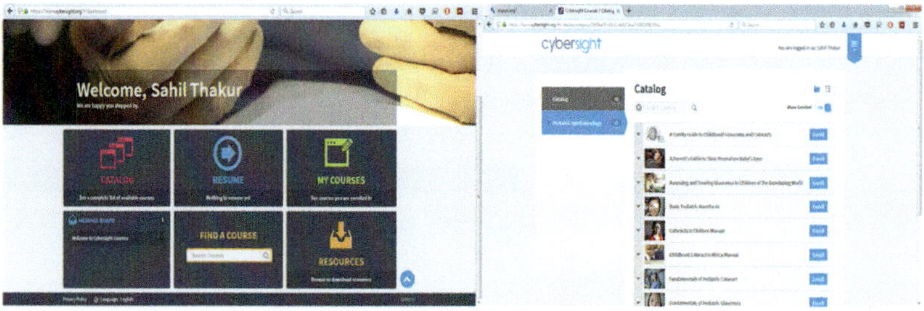

Site URL: https://cybersight.org/

B. ***Facebook Pages***

S. No	Page icon	Page name	Description	QR code
POS Society pages				
1.	WSPOS	WSPOS	Official page of the WSPOS	
2.	aapos American Association for Pediatric Ophthalmology and Strabismus	AAPOS4kids	Official page of the AAPOS	
Physician information and training				
1.	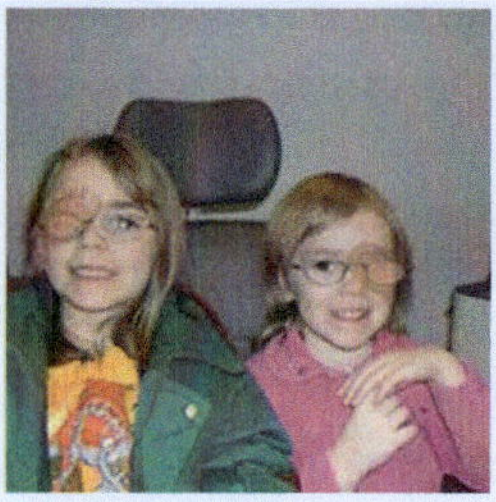	Paediatric Ophthalmology International Forum	This is a platform for residents and clinicians to share resources for education and training purposes	

S. No	Page icon	Page name	Description	QR code
2.		Paediatric Eye Doctors	This page regularly posts information regarding updates in the subspeciality	
3.	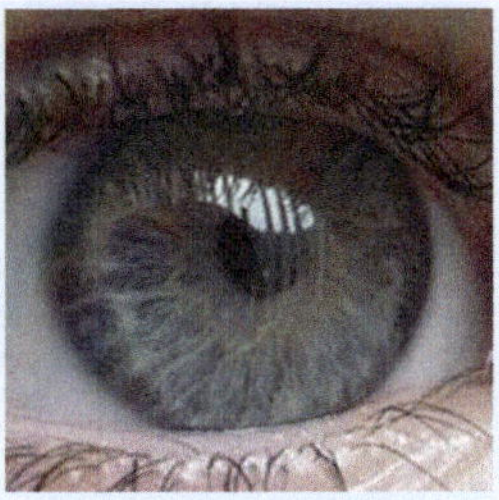	Strabismus	This page regularly posts squint cases and their management	
4.	Strabismus World	Strabismus World	This page regularly posts squint cases and their management	
Patient Support Groups				
1.	A MB LYOPIA KIDS.COM Amblyopia Kids Support Network www.amblyopiakids.com	AmblyopiaKids	This account promotes amblyopia awareness	
2.	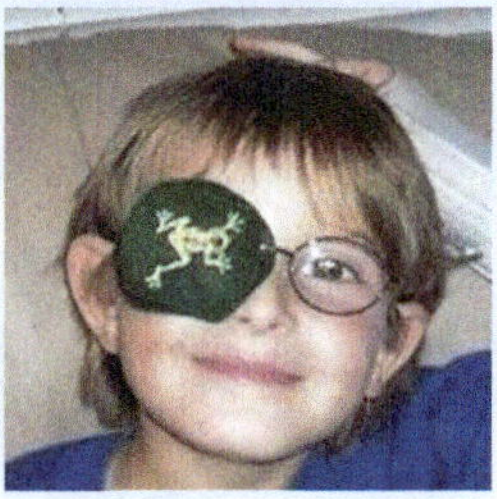	Amblyopia Support	This account promotes amblyopia awareness	

(continued)

S. No	Page icon	Page name	Description	QR code
3.		Children's Ptosis Foundation	Official page of the Ptosis Foundation	
4.		SeeVividly	Official page of the Vivid Vision company	

C. ***Twitter Handles***

S. No	Handle icon	Handle name	Description	QR code
1.		Aapos4kids	Official account of AAPOS	
2.		WSPOS	Official account of WSPOS	
3.	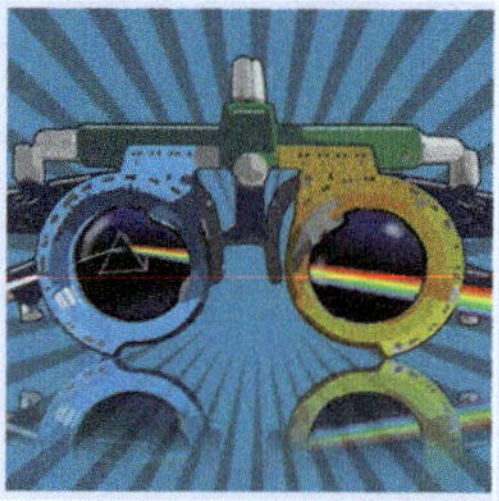	FollowIOA	Official account of the International Orthoptics Association	

S. No	Handle icon	Handle name	Description	QR code
4.		JPOS Journal	Official account of JPOS Journal	
5.		childrenseyefou	Official account of the Children's Eye Foundation	
6.	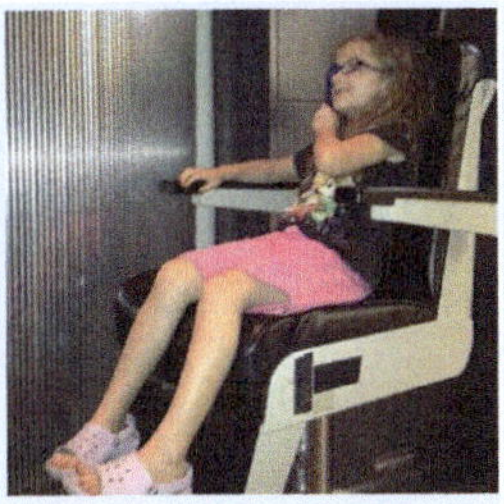	AmblyopiaKids	This account promotes amblyopia awareness	

References

1. Dahlmann-Noor A, Tailor V, Bunce C, Abou-Rayyah Y, Adams G, Brookes J, et al. Quality of Life and functional vision in children with glaucoma. Ophthalmology. 2017;124(7):1048–55.
2. Tsirlin I, Colpa L, Goltz HC, Wong AMF. Behavioral training as new treatment for adult amblyopia: a meta-analysis and systematic review. Invest Ophthalmol Vis Sci. 2015;56(6):4061–75.
3. Zhang JY, Cong LJ, Klein SA, Levi DM, Yu C. Perceptual learning improves adult amblyopic vision through rule-based cognitive compensation. Invest Ophthalmol Vis Sci. 2014;55(4):2020–30.
4. Hess RF, Thompson B, Black JM, Machara G, Zhang P, Bobier WR, et al. An iPod treatment of amblyopia: an updated binocular approach. Optometry. 2012;83(2):87–94.
5. To L, Thompson B, Blum JR, Maehara G, Hess RF, Cooperstock JR. A game platform for treatment of amblyopia. IEEE Trans Neural Syst Rehabil Eng. 2011;19(3):280–9.
6. Li RW, Ngo C, Nguyen J, Levi DM. Video-Game Play Induces Plasticity in the Visual System of Adults with Amblyopia. PLoS Biol. 2011;9(8):e1001135.

7. Kelly KR, Jost RM, Dao L, Beauchamp CL, Leffler JN, Birch EE. Binocular iPad game vs patching for treatment of amblyopia in children: a randomized clinical trial. JAMA Ophthalmol. 2016;134(12):1402–8.
8. Holmes JM, Manh VM, Lazar EL, Beck RW, Birch EE, Kraker RT, et al. Effect of a binocular iPad game vs part-time patching in children aged 5 to 12 years with amblyopia: a randomized clinical trial. JAMA Ophthalmol. 2016;134(12):1391–400.
9. Gargantini A, Terzi F, Zambelli M, Bonfanti S. A low-cost virtual reality game for amblyopia rehabilitation. In: Proceedings of the 3rd 2015 workshop on ICTs for improving patients rehabilitation research techniques, Lisbon, Portugal 2838964, ACM; 2015. pp. 81–4.
10. Mediklinik U. 2015 [cited 2017]. https://www.uvea.sk/en/news/item/554-virtualna-realita-funguje-prve-vysledky-liecby-tupozrakosti-na-slovensku%C2%A0
11. Aziz S, Cleary M, Stewart HK, Weir CR. Are orthoptic exercises an effective treatment for convergence and fusion deficiencies? Strabismus. 2006;14(4):183–9.
12. Petrunak JL. The treatment of convergence insufficiency. Am Orthopt J. 1999;49:12–6.

Apps and Social Networking Pages for Neuro-ophthalmology

8

Neuro-ophthalmology is one subspeciality that has always been an enigma for most practising ophthalmologists. The academic prowess of neuro-ophthalmologists is shown by the fact that the first four winners of the prestigious Straatsma American Academy of Ophthalmology teaching awards were all neuro-ophthalmologists [1]. However this academic-oriented branch demands high levels of patience and patient interaction that can often lead to frustration. This chapter aims to highlight some smartphone applications and web resources that can aid examination, help localize lesions and allow the neuro-ophthalmologist to do what they do best: unravel secrets beyond the optic nerve.

Applications

The apps have been discussed under the following heads:

A. Anatomy aids
B. Examination aids
C. Physician reference

A. **Anatomy Aids**
   1. ***Neuro Localizer HD***
      - ***Platforms: iOS iPad only***
      - ***App Creator: The University of Michigan***
      - ***Version: 1.1***
      - ***App Size: 8.7 MB***

P. Ichhpujani, S. Thakur, *Smart Resources in Ophthalmology*, Current Practices in Ophthalmology, https://doi.org/10.1007/978-981-13-0140-7_8

- ***App Icon:***

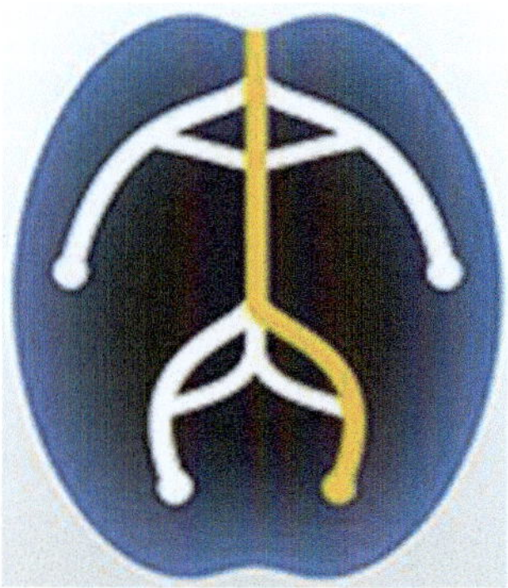

- ***App Screenshots:***

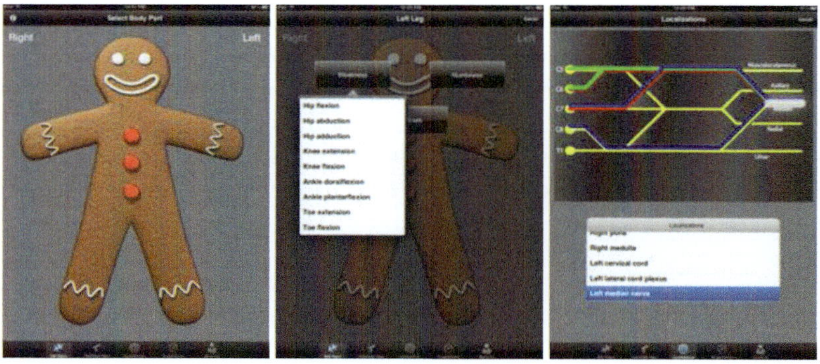

- ***Features:***
  This application provides a gingerbread man to mimic the patient's neurologic deficits. The 'Neuro Localize' helps in localizing the lesion. The user enters the symptoms or the abnormal findings of the exam, and the app draws the neuroanatomic pathways. The user can add information such as which muscles are weak, the location of numbness, any abnormal eye movements, which reflexes are brisk or hypoactive, etc. As more signs are added, Neuro Localizer shows where the pathways overlap in the central or peripheral nervous system. On the lighter side, the application can also give some life advice or tell a really great joke about gingerbread cookies and/or neurologists.

QR Scanning Codes for the App

2. ***Neuro AN***
   - ***Platforms: iOS (iPhone, iPad, iPod Touch)***
   - ***App Creator: Anatomy Next***
   - ***Version: 0.2***
   - ***App Size: 74.6 MB***
   - ***App Icon:***

   - ***App Screenshots:***

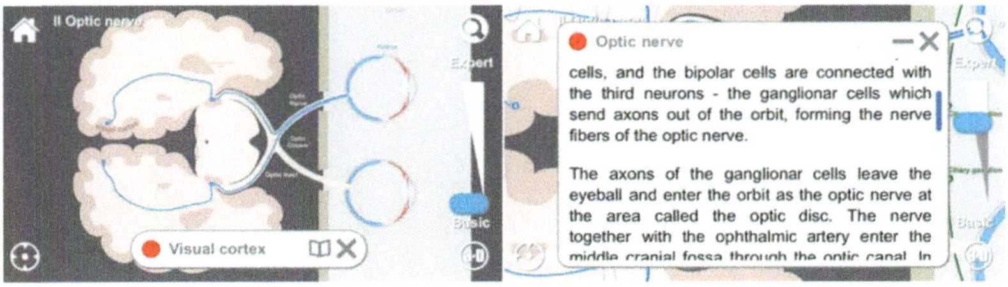

- ***Features:***
  This application is a complete guide to the anatomy of the cranial nerves. It is a combination of high-quality, easy-to-understand, interactive materials using accurate 3D models. There is availability of a combination of different cuts – sagittal, coronal and transverse. These 3D head and neck models can be viewed 360° in every plane of section to make every branch of every nerve and every structural detail ready for exploration. This application makes learning easier and more precise.

  QR Scanning Codes for the App

B. **Examination Aids**
   1. ***MRF Neural ($19.99)***
      - ***Platforms: iOS iPad only***
      - ***App Creator: Glance Optical Pty Ltd.***
      - ***Version: 1.0***
      - ***App Size: 24.5 MB***
      - ***App Icon:***

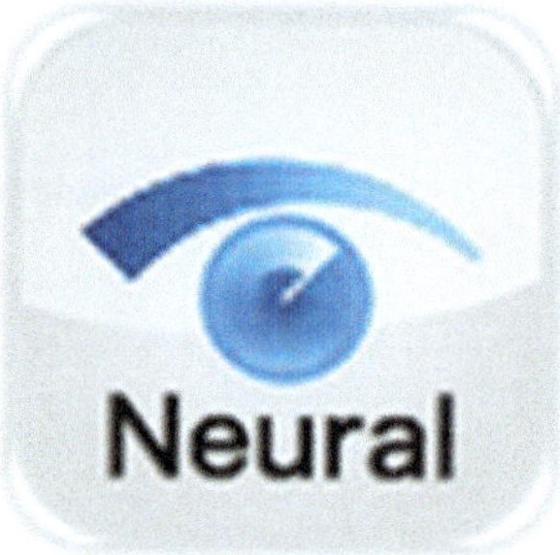

- ***App Screenshots:***

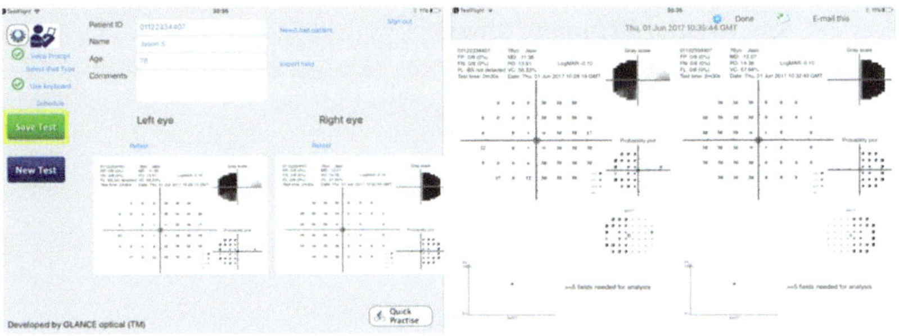

- ***Features:***
  This application provides a tool to evaluate problems in the visual field that occur in neurological conditions such as multiple sclerosis, optic neuritis, compressive optic neuropathy, pituitary lesion and stroke. MRF neurology has been designed to detect abnormalities in the visual field both centrally and in the periphery found in patients with neurological conditions. It offers full threshold testing up to 24° from fixation and vision monitoring. Longitudinal comparison of test results is performed at the end of each test. Test results are stored and can be accessed through an online portal. Test results can be exported as comma-separated values (.CVS) format and imported into Excel for detailed point-to-point analysis (for vision research purpose).

  Recently the role of tablet-based perimetry for assessment of bed-bound patients of tumours that compress the optic chiasm, like haemangiopericytoma, has been demonstrated successfully [2].

QR Scanning Codes for the App

2. ***OKN Strips ($2.99)***
   - ***Platforms: iOS***
   - ***App Creator: Thomas Alvarez***
   - ***Version: 1.3.1***
   - ***App Size: 1.2 MB***
   - ***App Icon:***

   - ***App Screenshots:***

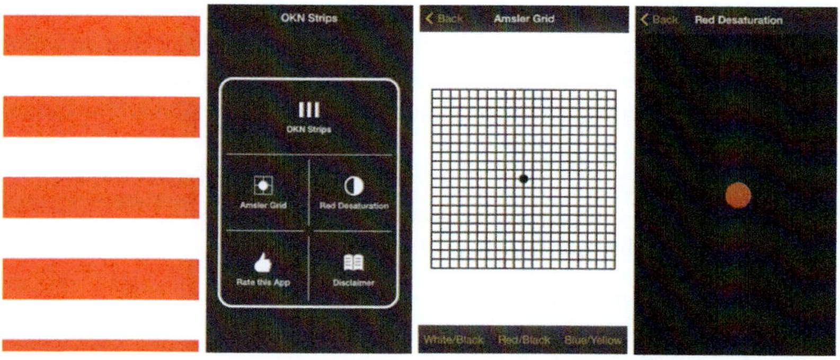

   - ***Features:***

   This application can be used to elicit optokinetic nystagmus (OKN) for evaluation of ophthalmological, neurological or otological disorders. The optokinetic response is a combination of slow-phase and fast-phase eye movements. It is seen when an individual follows a moving object with their eyes, which then moves out of the field of vision at which point their eye moves back to the position it was in when it first saw the object. It has been shown to help assess visual function in visually impaired patients [3]. The application includes a red desaturation mode and an Amsler grid for additional eye testing.

QR Scanning Codes for the App

3. ***Visual Fields Easy***
   - ***Platforms***: iOS (iPad only)
   - ***App Creator***: George Kong Softwares
   - ***Version***: 8.1
   - ***App Size***: 16.1 MB
   - ***App Icon***:

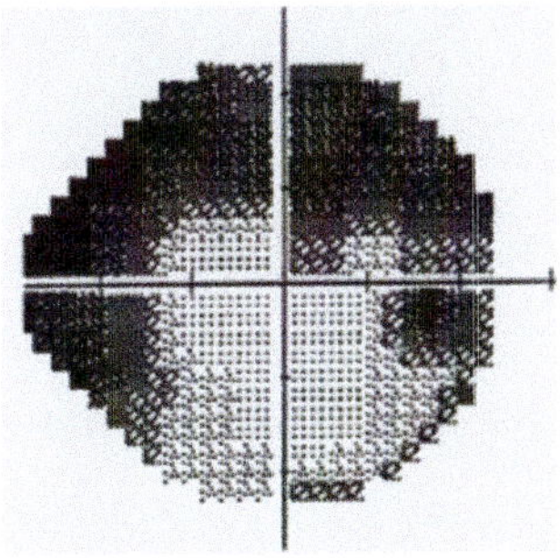

   - ***App Screenshot***:

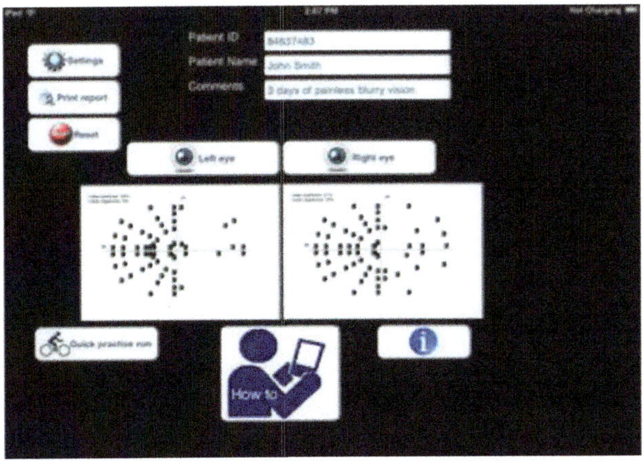

- ***Features***:
  This application uses the suprathreshold method of visual fields testing to detect gross abnormalities in the visual fields. The application offers a simple and fast way for visual field assessment but has been superseded by Melbourne Rapid Fields (MRF) application that provides better data for comparative assessment with the conventional Humphrey visual fields. Recently published data shows that as a screening tool for patients of stroke, the VFE application is easy to administer and preferred by patients and has good sensitivity and specificity for detecting the presence of an abnormal visual field when compared to white-on-white Humphrey visual field (HVF). In patients with advanced visual field damage, the VFE may however overestimate visual field reduction as compared to HVF [4].

  QR Scanning Code for the App

C. **Physician Reference**
   1. ***Neuro Board Review (In app purchase for sub speciality starting $29.99)***
      - ***Platforms***: iOS
      - ***App Creator***: Colen Publishing
      - ***Version***: 1.6
      - ***App Size***: 8.9 MB
      - ***App Icon***:

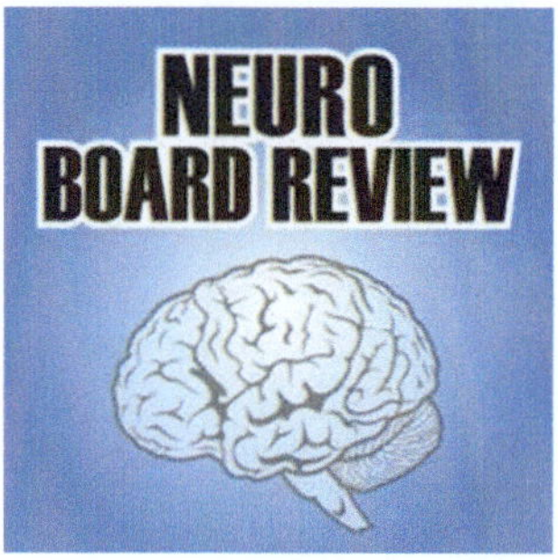

- ***App Screenshots***:

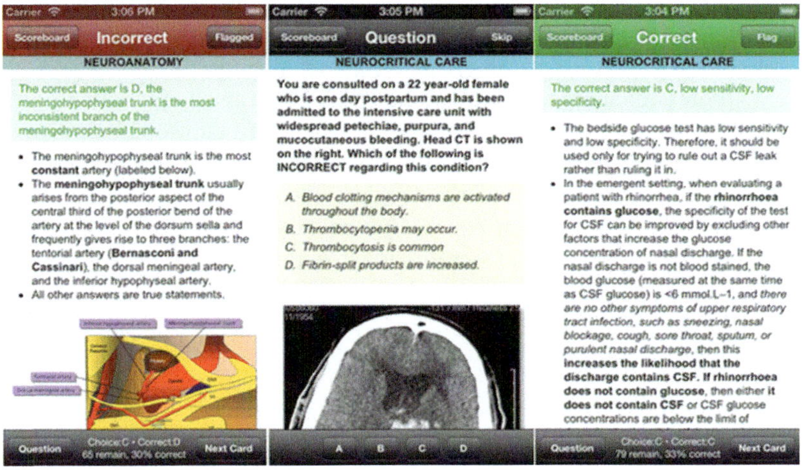

- ***Features***:
  The information pool for neuroanatomy, neurology and neuro-ophthalmology is increasing both in scope and complexity, and the current day clinicians often find it difficult to keep abreast with the vast knowledge base. This flashcard-based application can be used for quick access while in wards to practice the art of making a diagnosis. These cards are not the substitutes for standard comprehensive texts and atlases, but are a great way to refresh the information learned from the bedside, operating room and standard books.

  QR Scanning Codes for the App

Social Networking

A. ***Web Resources***

1. ***NANOS***: The North American Neuro-Ophthalmology Society (NANOS) is a professional organization of more than 600 trained ophthalmologists or neurologists. This society promotes the field of neuro-ophthalmology by supporting all forms of education, encouraging research and fostering clinical expertise. NANOS and its members sponsor an annual scientific meeting, publish the *Journal of Neuro-Ophthalmology*, recognize young researchers, contribute to numerous professional seminars and provide an email discussion list for lively clinical exchanges, NANOSNET.

   Website Screenshots

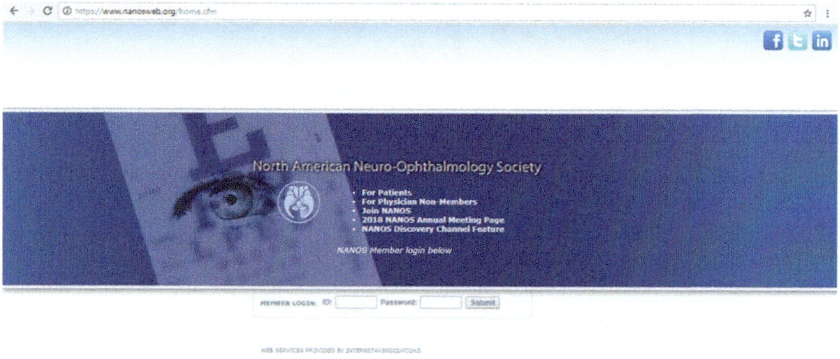

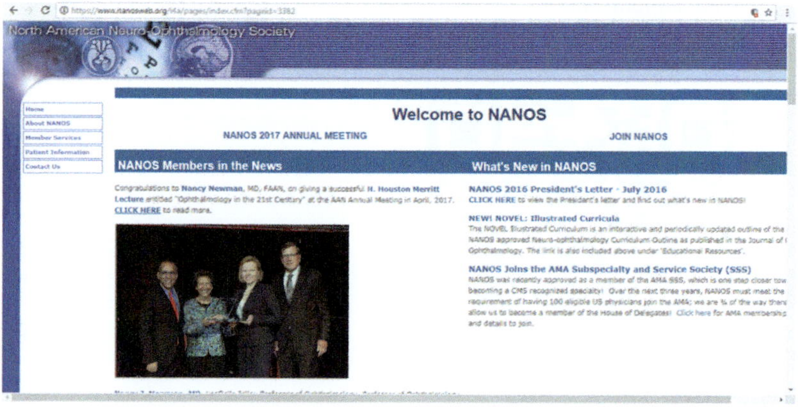

   Site URL: *https://www.nanosweb.org*

2. ***Canadian Neuro-Ophthalmology Group***: This website has everything that a budding neuro-ophthalmologist requires. From downloadable lectures to case discussions, this is a one-stop resource for finding the best material out there for neuro-ophthalmology exam preparation.

Website Screenshots

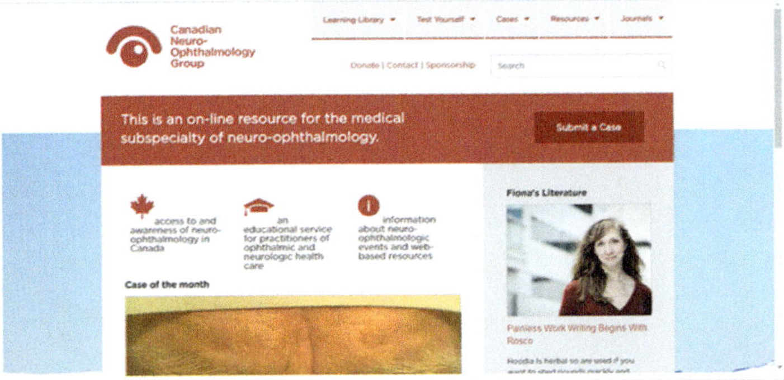

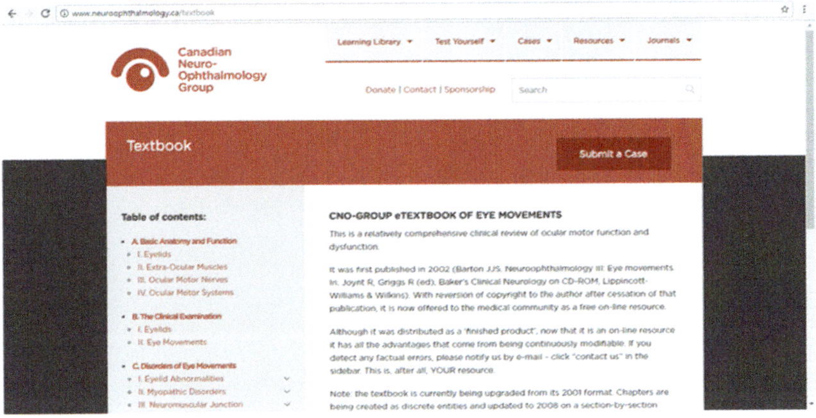

Site URL: *http://www.neuroophthalmology.ca/*

3. ***Journal of Neuro-Ophthalmology***: This is the official journal of the North American Neuro-Ophthalmology Society. The journal publishes salient advances in all spheres of the neurologic and ophthalmologic sciences. It has updates on recent developments in diagnosing and treating ophthalmologic, neurologic, endocrine, inflammatory and neoplastic conditions affecting the oculomotor and visual systems.

Website Screenshots

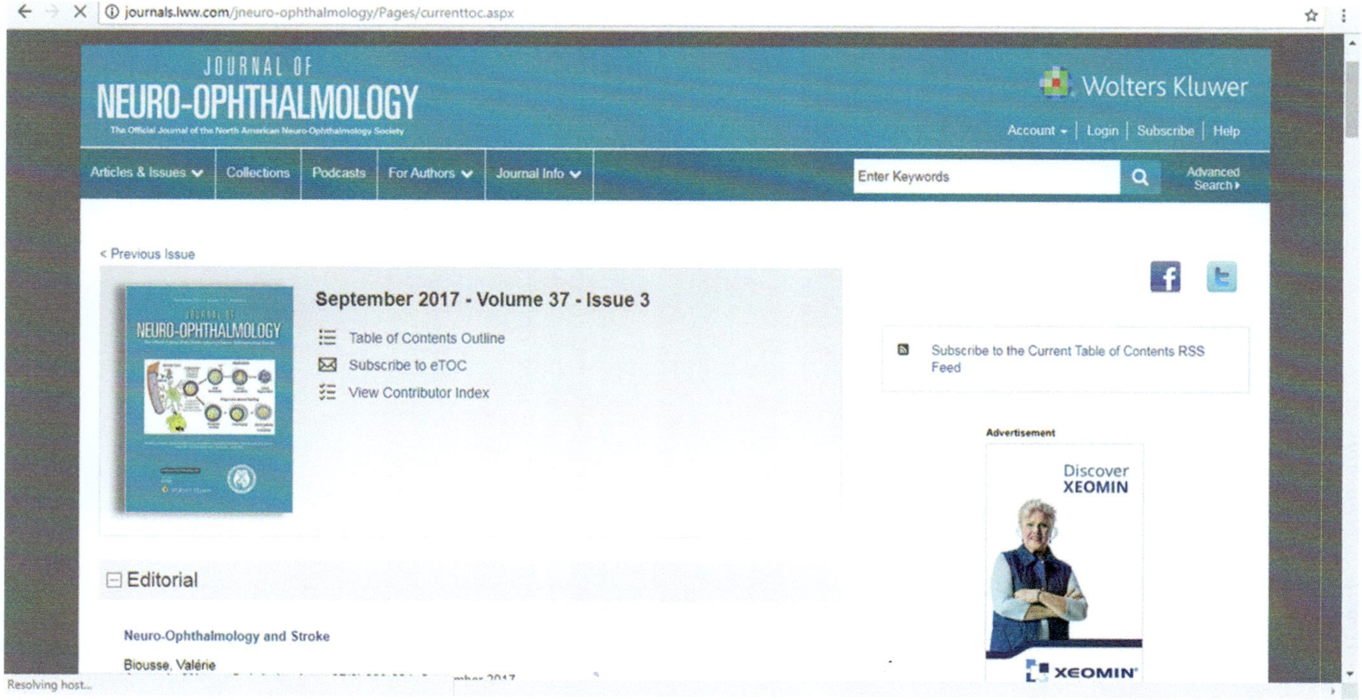

Site URL: *http://journals.lww.com/jneuro-ophthalmology/pages/default.aspx*

4. ***The Neuro-Ophthalmology Virtual Education Library (NOVEL)***
   NOVEL is a useful resource for learning neuro-ophthalmology, which is backed by NANOS and hosted by the University of Utah. It helps ophthalmologists in finding patient handouts and resources about neuro-ophthalmology. Dr. Neil Miller, chief editor of *Walsh and Hoyt's Clinical Neuro-Ophthalmology*, has generously provided the copyright license for distribution so that the entire textbook, all three volumes, are available for free download in PDF format. There are links to special collections containing lectures, images, articles, etc., from very distinguished and illustrious ophthalmologists and neuro-ophthalmologists. Manuscripts submitted to the *Journal of Neuro-Ophthalmology* and NOVEL are also available. There is a great patient portal that has NANOS-supported patient handouts covering many common neuro-ophthalmic conditions.

   Website Screenshot:

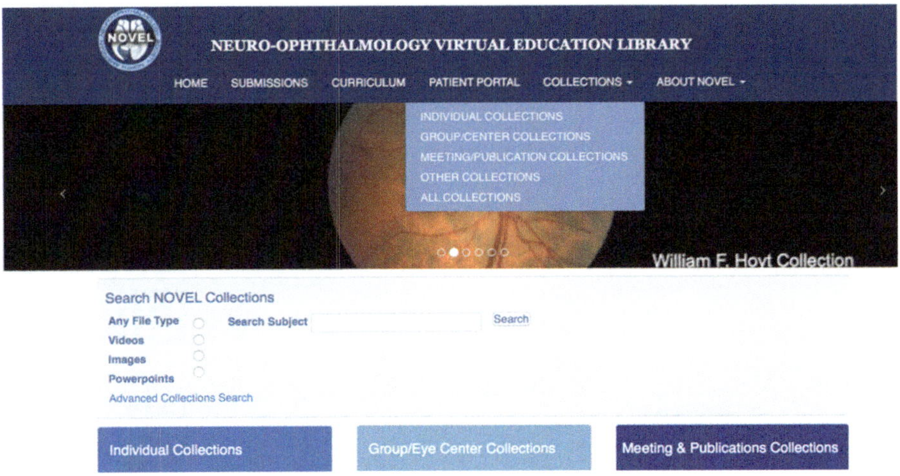

   Site URL: https://novel.utah.edu

B. ***Facebook Pages***

S. No	Page icon	Page name	Description	QR code
1.	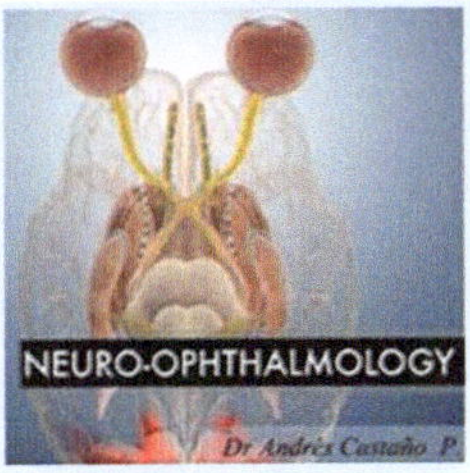	Neuro-ophthalmology	This page shares clinical vignettes, case reports and information about conferences that focus on neuro-ophthalmology	

S. No	Page icon	Page name	Description	QR code
2.	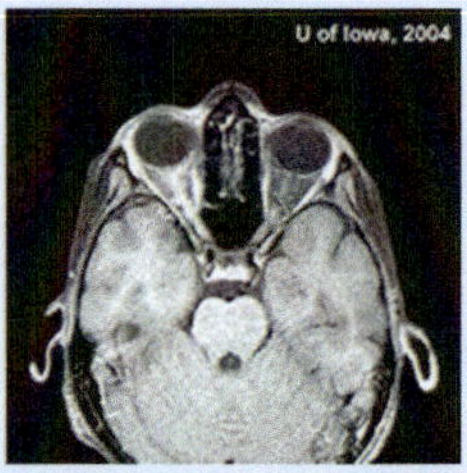	Neuro-Ophthalmology International Forum	Under the AAO, YO programme, this platform fosters international exchange of ideas and networking for eye care providers	
3.	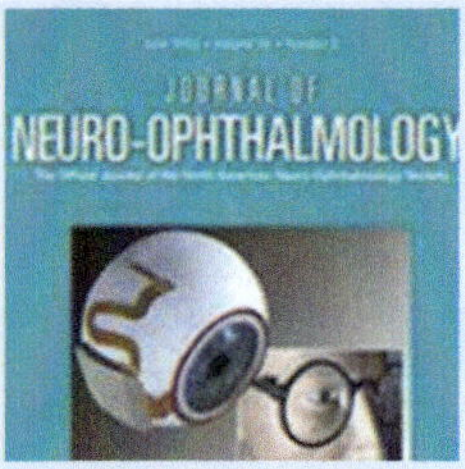	Journal of Neuro-Ophthalmology	Official journal of the North American Neuro-Ophthalmology Society	
4.	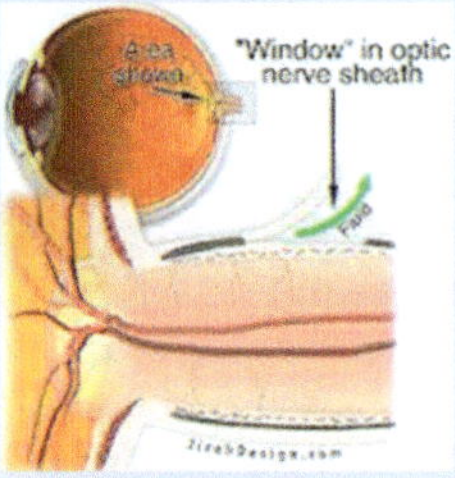	Neuro-ophthalmology Today	The page keeps you updated about the latest developments in the field of neurology and vision science	
5.	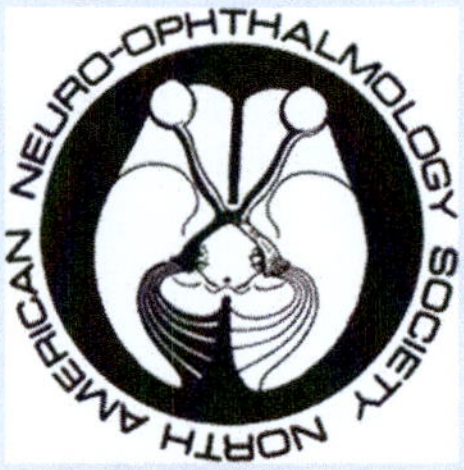	NANOS	The world's largest association of neuro-ophthalmologists dedicated to supporting neuro-ophthalmic patient care, clinical expertise, education and research	

C. ***Twitter Handles***

1.	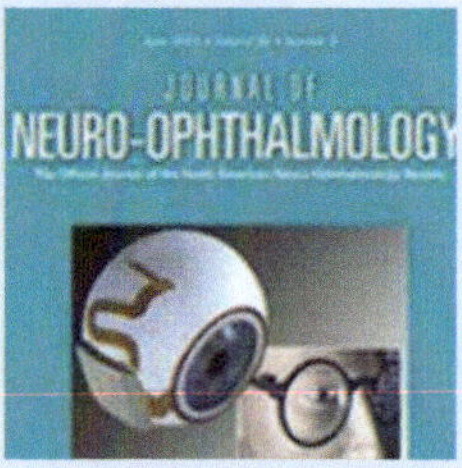	Journal of Neuro-Ophthalmology	Official journal of the North American Neuro-Ophthalmology Society	

So, learning neuro-ophthalmology can be fun with smartphones because of their inbuilt accelerometers that can be programmed to simulate a variety of eye movement and examples of pupillary reactions. Webpages and social media tools also lend a hand in making clinical neuro-ophthalmology principles user friendly and practical.

References

1. Frohman LP. The human resource crisis in neuro-ophthalmology. J Neuroophthalmol. 2008;28(3):231–4.
2. Nesaratnam N, Thomas PBM, Kirollos R, Vingrys AJ, Kong GYX, Martin KR. Tablets at the bedside—iPad-based visual field test used in the diagnosis of Intrasellar Haemangiopericytoma: a case report. BMC Ophthalmol. 2017;17(1):53.
3. Wester ST, Rizzo JF III, Balkwill MD, Wall C III. Optokinetic nystagmus as a measure of visual function in severely visually impaired patients. Invest Ophthalmol Vis Sci. 2007;48(10):4542–8.
4. Spofforth J, Codina C, Bjerre A. Is the 'visual fields easy' application a useful tool to identify visual field defects in patients who have suffered a stroke? Ophthalmol Res. 2017;7(1):1–10.

Apps and Social Networking Pages for Ocular Oncology, Oculoplasty and Ocular Trauma

9

The superspeciality of ocular oncology is focused on a diverse spectrum of ocular tumours, including lymphoma, retinoblastoma, adenoid cystic carcinoma, squamous cell carcinoma and melanoma. Across the globe, retinoblastoma remains the fatal paediatric ocular tumour.

Oculoplastics is the ophthalmic subspeciality that addresses examination, diagnosis and treatment of disorders, anomalies and injuries of the eyelids, lacrimal apparatus and the orbit. This includes pre- and postoperative evaluation and surgical management of oculoplastic and orbital disorders. Ocular trauma may need oculoplastic intervention for restoration of anatomy.

Applications

There are not many applications addressing the subspecialities of ocular oncology, oculoplasty and ocular trauma. The few that we could find have been divided under the following heads:

A. Applications to detect white eye reflex
B. Applications for clinical photography
C. Applications for scoring ocular trauma

A. **Applications to Detect White Eye Reflex**
   Retinoblastoma is the only ophthalmic tumour for which smartphone-based screening apps exist.
   1. **White Eye Detector (CRADLE White Eye Detector)**
      - ***Platforms***: iOS (iPhone and iPad); Android
      - ***App Creator***: Gregory Hamerly
      - ***Version*****:** 1.1 (English and Spanish)
      - ***App Size*****:** 6 MB

P. Ichhpujani, S. Thakur, *Smart Resources in Ophthalmology*, Current Practices in Ophthalmology, https://doi.org/10.1007/978-981-13-0140-7_9

- ***App Icon***:

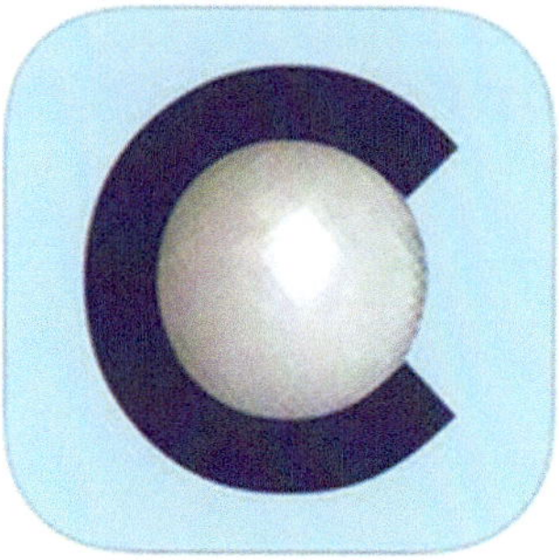

- ***App Screenshots***:

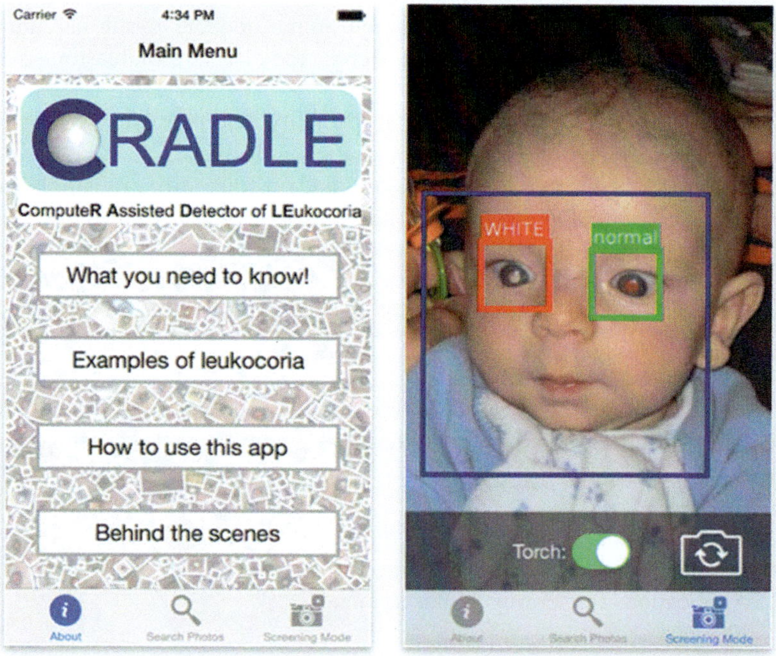

- ***Features***:
  CRADLE stands for ComputeR Assisted Detector of LEukocoria.
  CRADLE app was developed by an American engineer whose son's retinoblastoma was not diagnosed until he was 3 months old, even though photographs taken of him ever since he was 12 days old showed the white eye reflex.

The White Eye Detector app helps parents detect the appearance of white eye in photographs of their children. This app helps parents find pictures on their iPhone or iPad that have white, golden or a yellow glow. White eye can be a symptom of multiple serious eye diseases such as retinoblastoma, paediatric cataract and Coats' disease [1, 2].
The app can also be used in scanning mode by turning the smartphone into a crude ophthalmoscope and allowing the examiner to wave the device over the child's eyes. Green boxes appear around the eyes, and if a reflection is detected, the box turns red. This app may especially be useful for rapid leukocoria detection in resource-limited countries around the globe where ophthalmoscopes may not be available with the care providers.

- ***QR Scanning Code for the App***

iOS Android

2. **MD EyeCare**
   - ***Platforms***: iOS (iPhone and iPad)(English, Spanish)
   - ***App Creator***: Movidreams S.A
   - ***Version*: **1.1.1
   - ***App Size*: **26.6 MB
   - ***App Icon***:

- ***App Screenshots***:

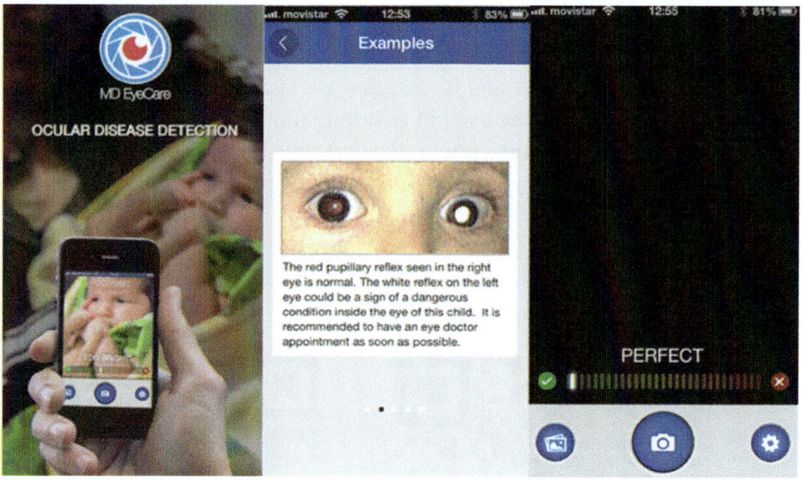

- ***Features***:

  MD EyeCare app was co-developed with Maria Manquez, an ocular oncologist, who is a member of the International Society of Ocular Oncology and part of the Eye Cancer Network. The app helps in taking a proper photograph of the eyes for early diagnosis of retinoblastoma in kids. It can serve as a low-cost screening tool for early diagnosis of the dreaded tumour.
  Note: Neither the White Eye Detector app nor the MD EyeCare app replaces the detailed medical examination by a trained ophthalmologist.
- ***QR Scanning Code for the App***

B. **Applications for Clinical Photography**
   Clinical photography in the field of oculoplastic surgery has many applications. Photographs are useful not only for clinical records, research and education but also as supportive evidence in medicolegal cases. Now, it is possible for clinicians to obtain high-quality clinical photographs using an app.

1. **IRISS Medigrid**

- ***Platforms***: iOS (iPhone and iPad)(USD74.99 per 3 months)
  - ***App Creator***: IRISS Medical
  - ***Version*****:** 1.23
  - ***App Size*****:** 26.6 MB
  - ***App Icon***:

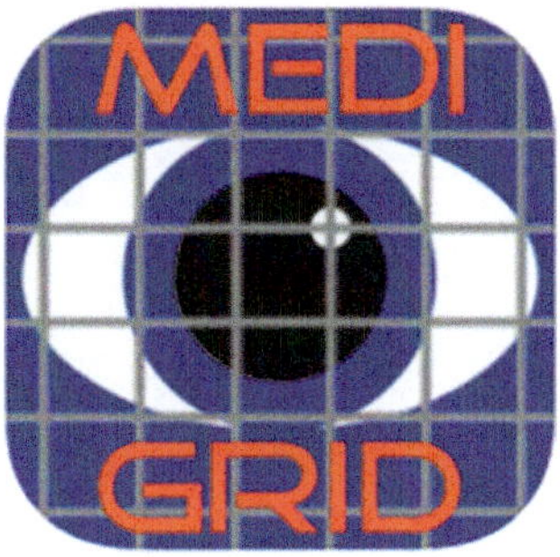

  - ***App Screenshots***:

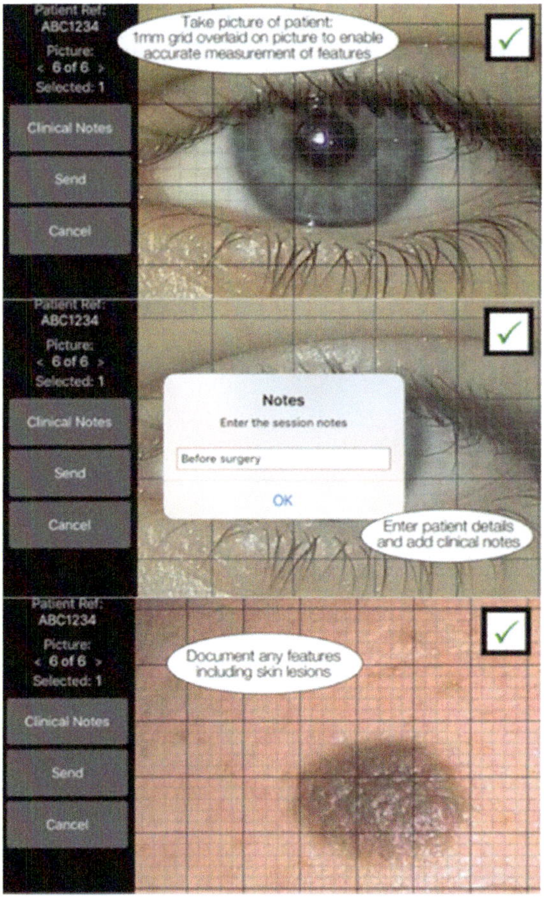

- ***Features***:
  This app is FDA cleared, CE Marked and HIPPA compliant. mediGrid enables physicians to measure and document any features on a patient's photo with an accuracy of 0.5 mm. It helps the physician record and save pre- and post-procedure (e.g. blepharoplasty) patient pictures. It allows for monitoring progress of a feature such as lesions, moles, etc.
- ***QR Scanning Code for the App***

C. **Applications for Scoring Ocular Trauma**
Classification systems are necessary to scientifically study the aetiology, pathogenesis and treatment of diseases in a uniform fashion. Many a times periocular soft tissue injuries involving the upper eyelid, lower eyelid and medial and lateral canthus are not recorded appropriately. A new app based on clinico-anatomical patterns of injuries has been designed to guide the ophthalmic and facial reconstructive surgeons to provide optimal outcomes in eyelid injuries.

1. **SPOT Eye APK**
   - ***Platforms***: Android
   - ***App Creator***: Prem Prakash Sahoo (JIPMER)
   - ***Version*****:** 0.0.3
   - ***App Icon***:

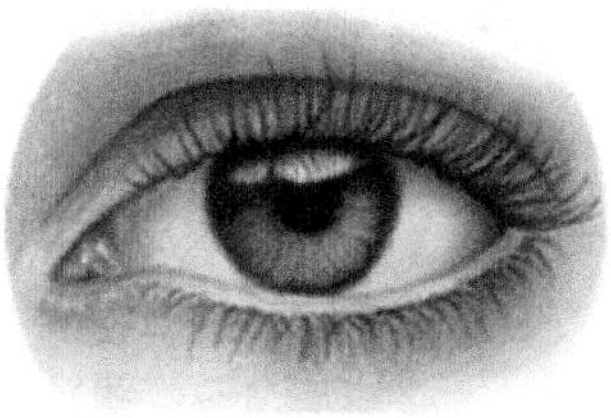

- ***App Screenshots***:

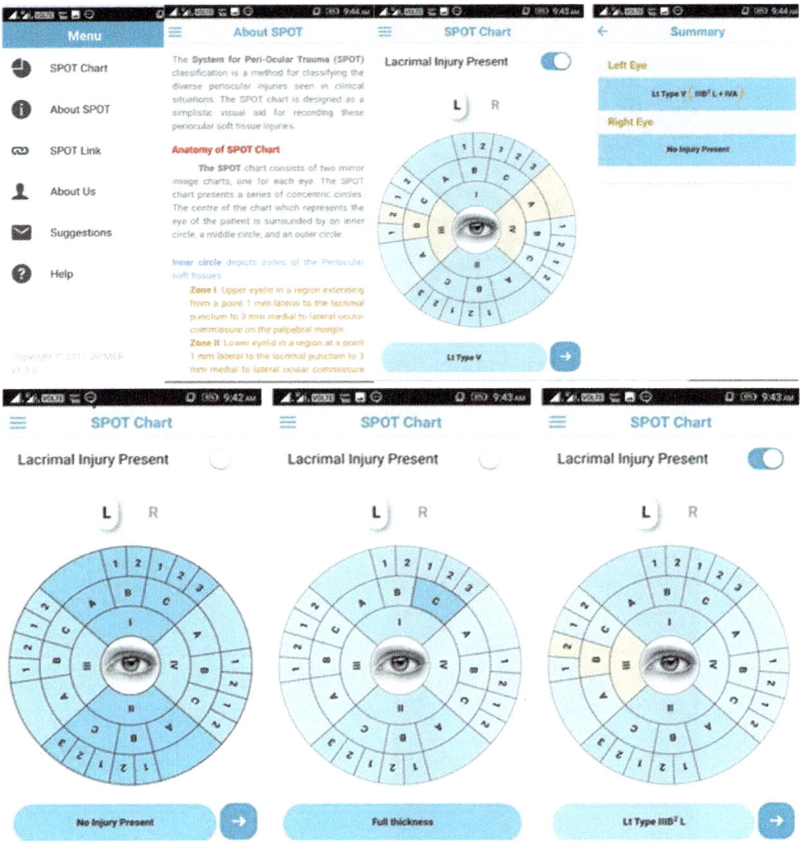

- ***Features***:
  The SPOT (System for Peri-Ocular Trauma) Eye app presents an interactive SPOT Chart for recording periocular injuries. It has been designed for medical and allied professionals who deal with eyelid injuries in their clinical practice. The app helps the observer identify and record the eyelid injuries of the patient according to the SPOT classification, which describes the periocular soft tissue injuries according to the location, severity and extent [3].

- ***QR Scanning Code of the App***

2. **Ocular Trauma Score Application**
   - ***Platforms***: Android
   - ***App Creator***: Pixelwyrm Studios
   - ***Version*:** 1.1
   - ***App Icon***:

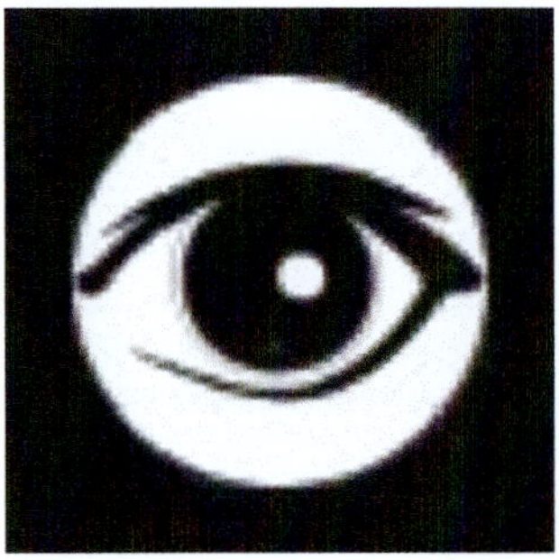

   - ***App Screenshots***:

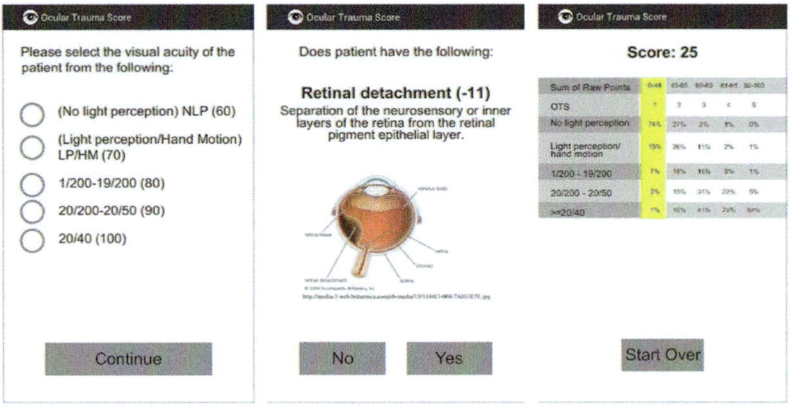

- ***Features***:

  The Ocular Trauma Score application allows physicians to predict visual acuity outcomes based on initial examination parameters after ocular trauma. The OTSA provides a user-friendly interface to input data points based on exam findings in a template manner to calculate their OTS. This application is available on the Dolphin Market and from the QR code below.

  QR Scanning Code of the App

Social Networking

A. ***Web Resources***

1. ***International Society of Ocular Oncology***

   The mission of the International Society of Ocular Oncology is to promote the advancement of ocular oncology by increasing coordination between general ophthalmology, general oncology, ophthalmic pathology and allied sciences. The society also encourages research and aids in the improvement of teaching and technical methods. Additionally, it contributes to improvement of patient care, through scientific meetings and other activities worldwide. The website offers a sneak peek into the history of the society and under the Resource section photographically enlists all the ocular tumours.

Website Screenshots:

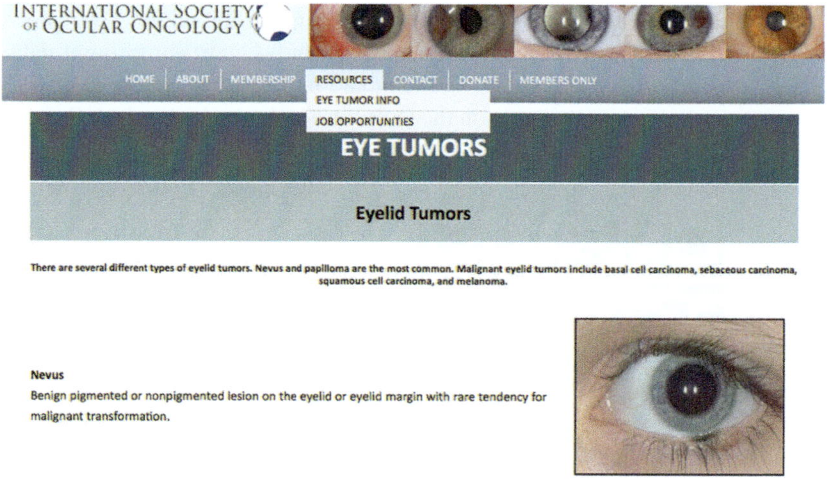

Site URL: http://www.isoo.org

2. ***Oculoplastic Association of India***
   This society serves as a link between the members interested in the speciality of oculoplastic, orbital and lacrimal disorders. The body not only promotes education, academic and research activities but also assists in the members of the association to achieve these goals. In addition to the society, conference and meeting information, the website offers an active discussion forum for the members to discuss challenging cases or share newer advances.

Website Screenshots:

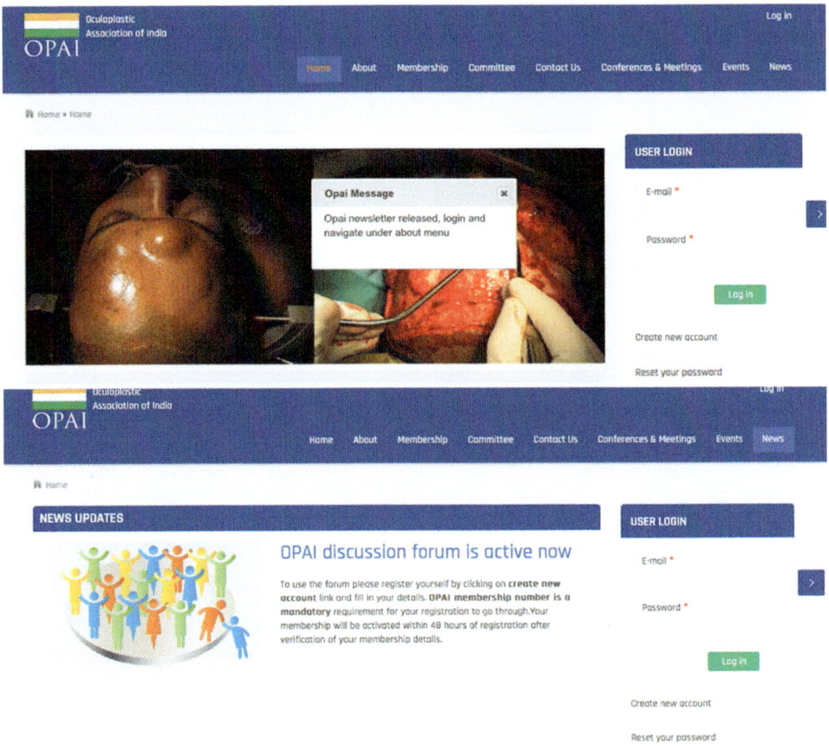

Site URL: http://www.opai.in

3. ***AAO Ocular Pathology/Oncology: One Network:*** It offers the best content on ocular oncology; however the multimedia content requires an AAO subscription. Still it is the best place to get the latest information about the subspeciality.

- **Website Screenshots:**

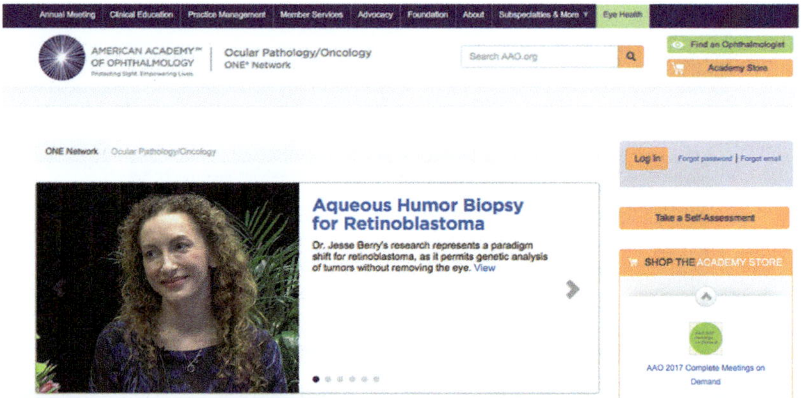

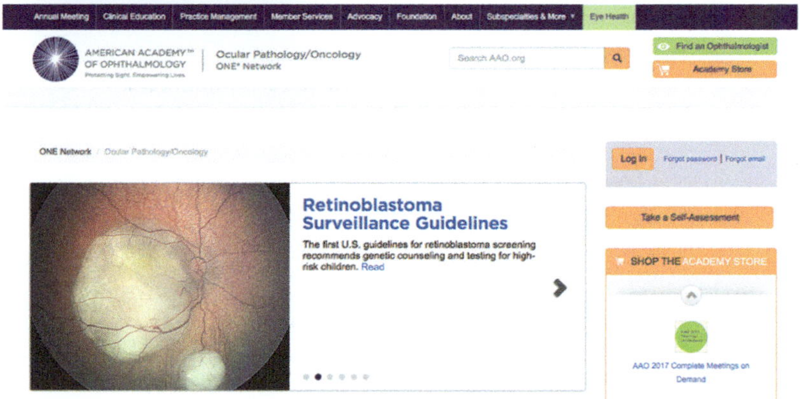

Site URL: https://www.aao.org/ocular-pathology-oncology

4. ***International Society of Oculoplastic and Reconstructive Surgeons (ISOPRS)***
   The society promotes an integrated approach for the treatment of orbital and ophthalmic injuries, ensuring the physician is able to provide the patient with the benefits of not only ophthalmology and plastic surgery but also neurology and ENT skills with a readily accessible knowledge base and understanding of basic pathology and radiology. The webpage also has a video section and a link to the society journal, *Journal of International Society of Oculoplastic and Reconstructive Surgeons*.

- ***Website Screenshot:***

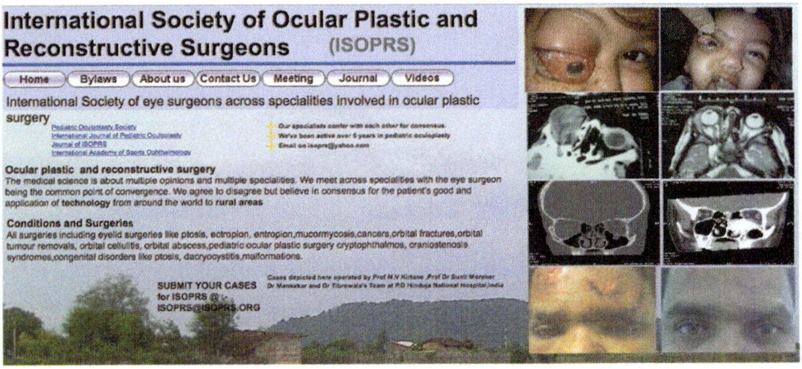

Site URL: http://www.isoprs.org

5. ***Melanoma Research Foundation (MRF)***

   MRF is the largest non-profit organization committed to the support of medical research in finding effective treatments and hopefully a cure for melanoma. The organization also educates patients, caregivers and physicians about the prevention, diagnosis and treatment of all types of melanoma including ocular melanoma.

   CURE OM (the **C**ommunity **U**nited for **R**esearch and **E**ducation of **O**cular **M**elanoma), founded in 2011, is the MRF's initiative on ocular melanoma to increase awareness, education, treatment and research funding for ocular melanoma.

- ***Website Screenshot:***

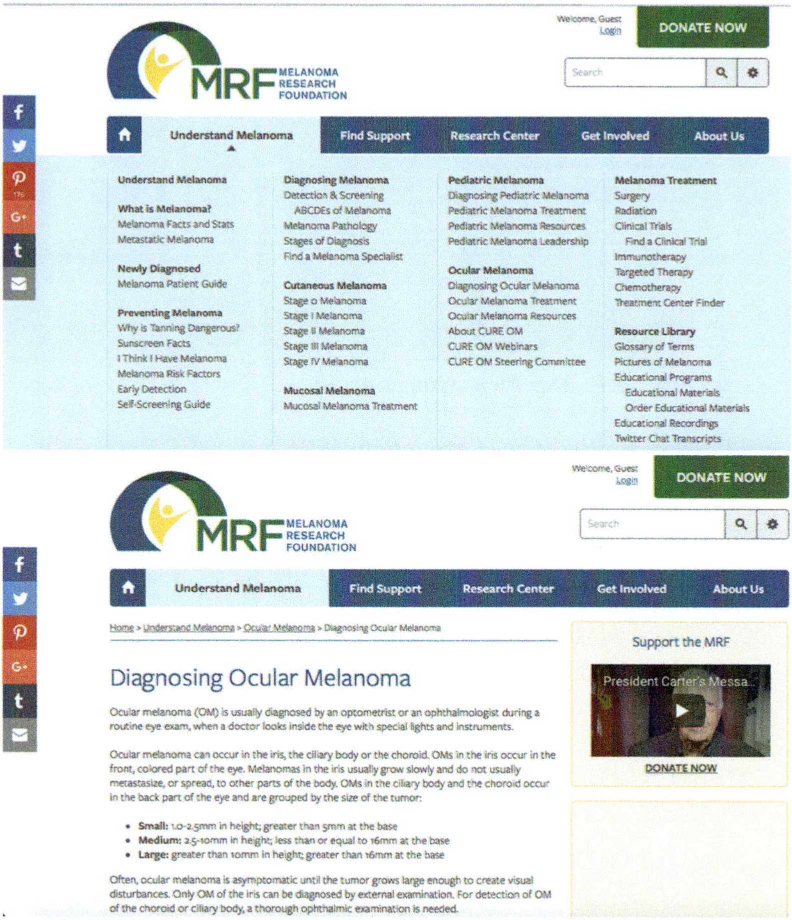

Website URL: https://www.melanoma.org

6. ***Ocular Trauma Society of India***
   Ocular Trauma Society of India aims to assimilate information, generate epidemiological data and develop uniform treatment protocols for ocular trauma in India. It is working to form a registry—a Pan-India database of ocular injuries, their nature, course and outcomes.

- ***Website Screenshots:***

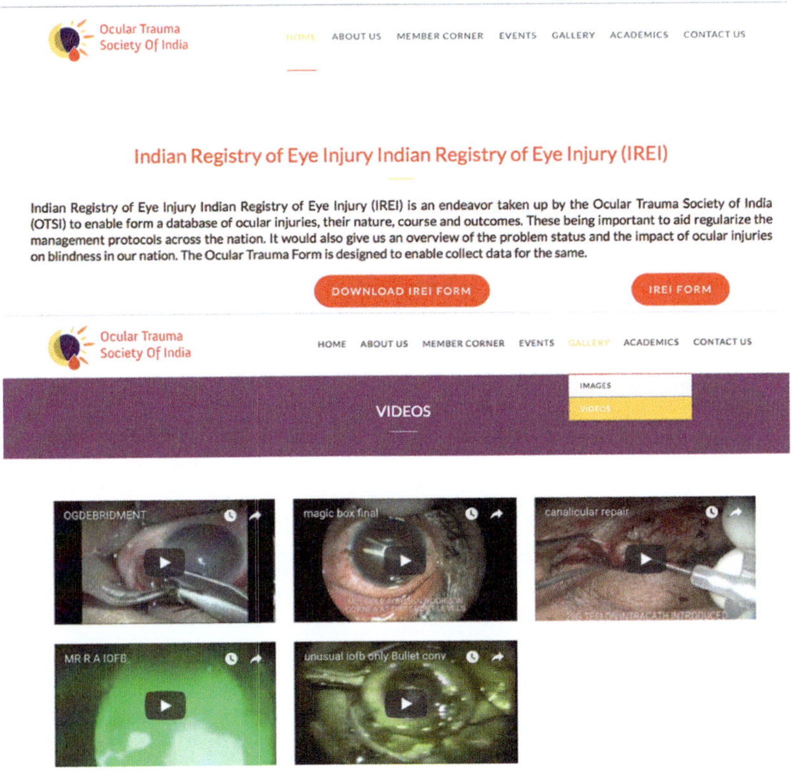

Site URL: http://www.otsi.in

7. ***CANKIDS***
   CANKIDS is a grassroot-level organization of over 300 individuals (volunteers as well as employees) that works on all aspects to enable best standards of treatment care and support services for children with cancer and their families, from the time of diagnosis through treatment and even into survivorship. They also provide palliative care and terminal and bereavement support. The members are doing commendable work with patients of retinoblastoma.

- ***Website Screenshots:***

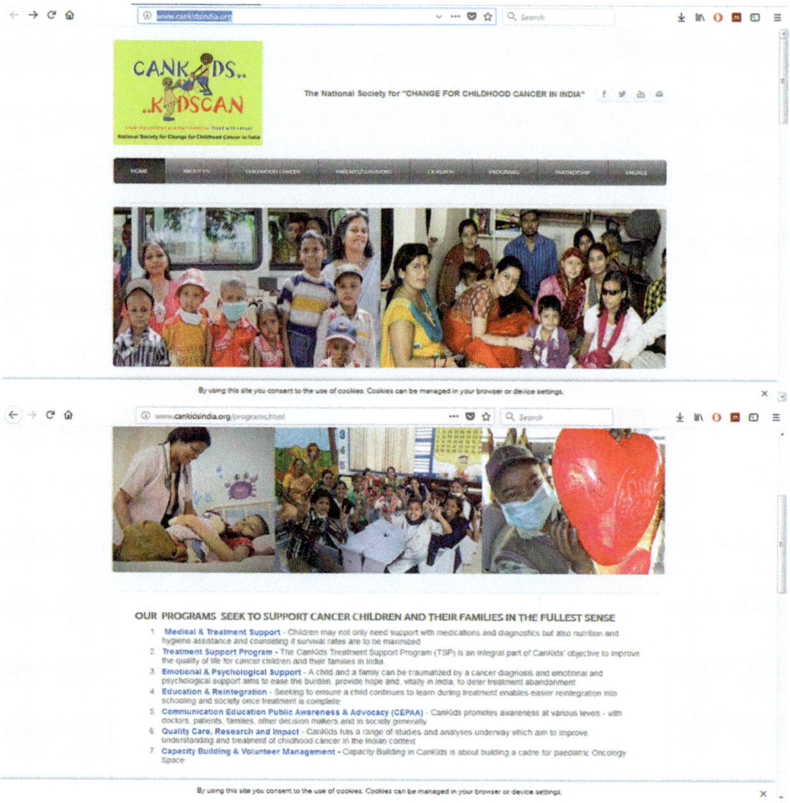

Site URL: http://www.cankidsindia.org/

8. **Atlas of Genetics and Cytogenetics in Oncology and Haematology: Eye Tumours**
   This is a very good resource for residents and fellows who struggle with ophthalmic pathology and intraocular tumours. Each major tumour is described in detail regarding aetiology, epidemiology, clinical presentation, pathology, cytogenetics/genes (when available), treatment options and prognosis.

- ***Website Screenshot:***

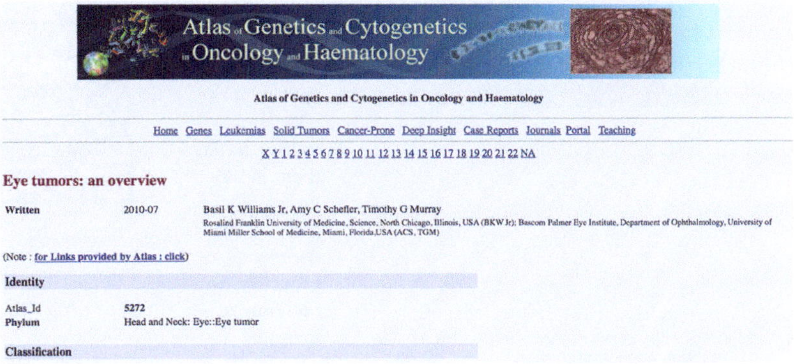

Atlas of Genetics and Cytogenetics in Oncology and Haematology

Atlas of Genetics and Cytogenetics in Oncology and Haematology

Home Genes Leukemias Solid Tumors Cancer-Prone Deep Insight Case Reports Journals Portal Teaching

X Y 1 2 3 4 5 6 7 8 9 10 11 12 13 14 15 16 17 18 19 20 21 22 NA

Eye tumors: an overview

Written	2010-07	Basil K Williams Jr, Amy C Schefler, Timothy G Murray Rosalind Franklin University of Medicine, Science, North Chicago, Illinois, USA (BKW Jr); Bascom Palmer Eye Institute, Department of Ophthalmology, University of Miami Miller School of Medicine, Miami, Florida,USA (ACS, TGM)

(Note : for Links provided by Atlas : click)

Identity

Atlas_Id	**5272**
Phylum	Head and Neck: Eye::Eye tumor

Classification

Site URL: http://atlasgeneticsoncology.org/Tumors/EyeTumOverviewID5272.html

B. ***Facebook Pages***

S. No	Page icon	Page name	Description	QR code
Society pages				
1.		***Asia Pacific Ophthalmic Trauma Society***	The official FB page of the society	
2.		***Ocular Trauma Society of India***	The official FB page of the ocular trauma society of India	

S. No	Page icon	Page name	Description	QR code
Patient support groups				
1.	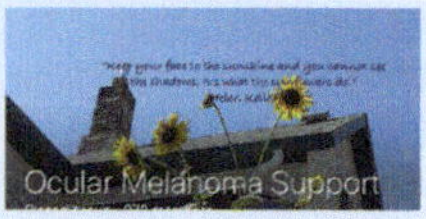	Ocular Melanoma Support	This is groups for patients and for their spouse, if the patient is willing to have them in the group. The patients share their experience and outcome of therapy	
2.	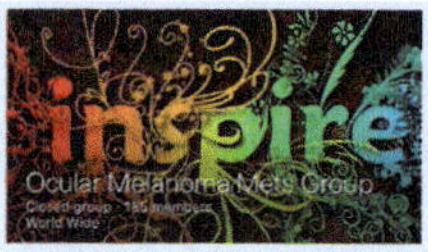	Ocular Melanoma Mets group	This group is reserved for those with metastatic ocular melanoma	
3.		Childhood Eye Cancer Trust (CHECT)	This is a UK charity dedicated to helping people affected by retinoblastoma and fund research into the prevention and treatment of RB	
4.	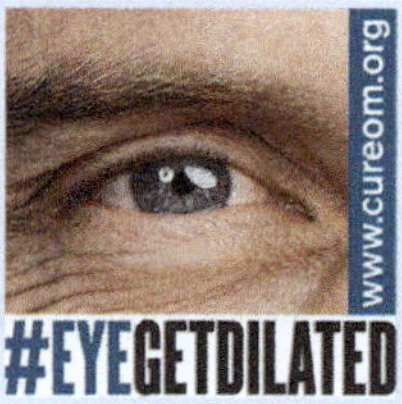	***CURE Ocular Melanoma***	CURE OM is MRF's initiative to increase awareness, education, treatment and research funding of ocular melanoma	

C. *Twitter Handles*

S. No	Handle icon	Handle name	Description	QR code
1.		Ocular Oncology @ LOOC_UK_ COM	It is the handle for The Liverpool Ocular Oncology Centre at the Royal Liverpool University Hospital. The handle helps patients with ocular tumours	
2.		CURE Ocular Melanoma @ MRFCureOM	It is the handle for the MRF's initiative to advance research and provide educational resources for ocular melanoma.	
3.		UM CURE 2020 @ UMCURE2020	This is the handle for a funded project for newer therapeutic approaches for metastatic uveal melanoma	
4.		World Eye Cancer Hope @wechope	This handle spreads awareness for paediatric ocular tumours. It also addresses medical care, family support and research	
5.		CRRAB @rb_research	This Canadian Retinoblastoma Research Advisory Board aims to research newer modalities to improve therapeutic outcome for retinoblastoma	

S. No	Handle icon	Handle name	Description	QR code
6.		Oculoplastic Surgery @ASOPRS	The American Society of Ophthalmic Plastic and Reconstructive Surgery aims to advance education, research and the practice of plastic and reconstructive surgery for the face, orbits, eyelids and lacrimal system	

These 'pot pourri' resources based on smart devices not only help to educate the doctors but also assure the caregivers that there are several avenues to ease the demands of the ocular tumours and trauma.

References

1. Haider S, Qureshi W, Ali A. Leukocoria in children. J Pediatr Ophthalmol Strabismus. 2008;45(3):179–80.
2. Abdolvahabi A, Taylor BW, Holden RL, Shaw EV, Kentsis A, et al. Colorimetric and longitudinal analysis of leukocoria in recreational photographs of children with retinoblastoma. PLoS One. 2013;8(10):e76677. https://doi.org/10.1371/journal.pone.0076677.
3. Mohapatra DP, Thiruvoth FM, Chittoria RK, Kumar SD, Kumar SH, Kumar S, et al. Proposal of a new classification scheme for periocular injuries. Indian J Plast Surg. 2017;50:21–8.

Apps for Data Mining

10

The past decade has seen the rise of the Internet as an indispensable source of information about health, diseases and medical treatment, for not only the healthy individuals and patients but also healthcare professionals. It has hence become a necessity for medical practitioners to actively engage in this huge network of data exchange. '*Publish or Perish*' has become the modern-day rule for the scientific community. Barjak studied the effect of Internet use on research productivity and demonstrated that the researchers, who were net savvy, communicated via email, used individual homepages (with full text) and electronic journals, published more journal articles than their peers who did not use the Internet-based tools [1]. It is thus imperative that we discuss tools that can make this data search more efficient. Data mining using mobile devices thus can effectively streamline your research methodology.

Applications

Offering portability, flexibility and ease of use, the applications that are discussed below can become your primary way of searching, recording and reproducing scientific data.

1. ***Medscape***
   - ***Platforms***: iOS and Android
   - ***App Creator***: WebMD
   - ***Version***: 4.0.3
   - ***App Size***: 27.1 MB

P. Ichhpujani, S. Thakur, *Smart Resources in Ophthalmology*, Current Practices in Ophthalmology, https://doi.org/10.1007/978-981-13-0140-7_10

- ***App Icon***:

- ***App Screenshots***:

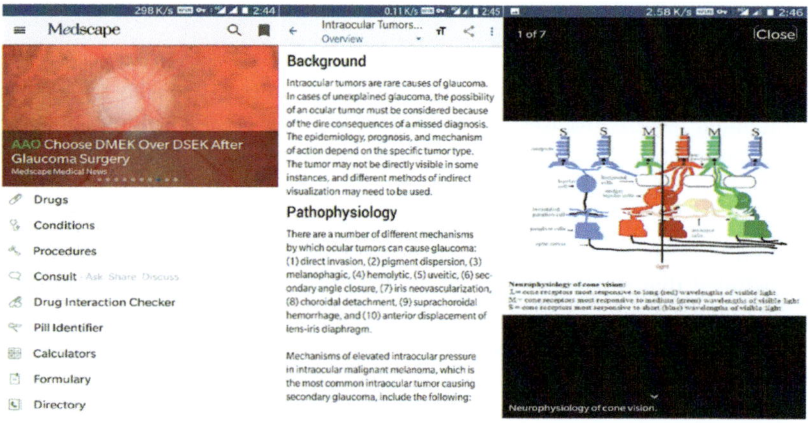

- ***Features***:
  This application is the leading medical resource for physicians, medical students, nurses and other healthcare professionals as it provides fast and accurate clinical answers at the point of care. It has sections to quickly look up medications and dosages with a Drug Reference Tool and Drug Interaction Checker. Other useful resources located within the app include medical calculators, pill ID tool, step-by-step procedural articles and collections of images. The application is free to use but a *Login* is required the first time. A free account can be made inside the app.

  QR Scanning Codes for the App

  Android

  iOS

2. ***Read by QxMD***
   - ***Platforms***: iOS and Android
   - ***App Creator***: QxMD
   - ***Version***: 6.12
   - ***App Size***: 39.1 MB
   - ***App Icon***:

   - ***App Screenshots***:

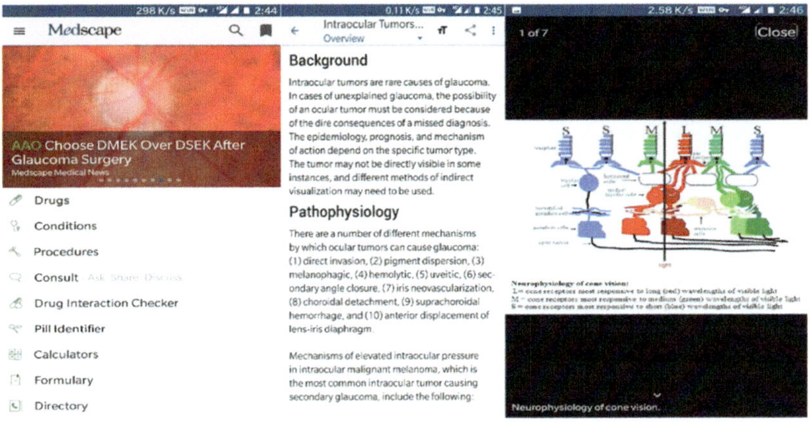

   - ***Features***:
     This free application helps the user to keep abreast with the latest medical and scientific research and search PubMed and provides outstanding topic reviews. The user can formulate a custom journal timeline. The app provides one touch access to pdfs, has an inbuilt pdf reader, provides access to full text via university/institutional subscription or open access publishers and allows for instant sharing on social media. These features make this application a must have for avid researchers.

QR Scanning Codes for the App

Android iOS

3. ***Prime: PubMed, Journals, and Grapherence® Access***
   - ***Platforms***: iOS and Android
   - ***App Creator***: Unbound Medicine
   - ***Version***: 2.2
   - ***App Size***: 7.5 MB
   - ***App Icon***:

- *App Screenshots*:

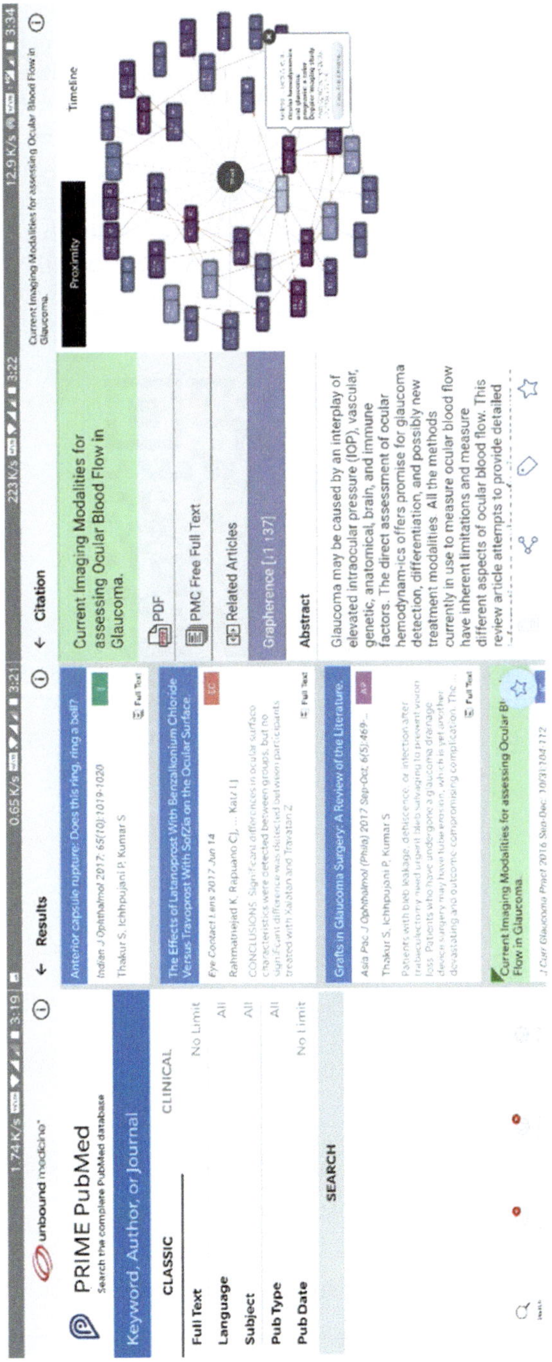

- ***Features***:
  This application is helpful in connecting to the most up-to-date journal citations and abstracts from the PubMed database. In addition to the ability to perform powerful searches and link to the publisher's full text articles, Prime also provides a number of exclusive tools not available anywhere else. Grapherence® is Unbound's interactive search that graphically represents the influence and interrelationships among journal articles. The Grapherence button within a citation allows the user to see how that article is related to others. This can aid in faster assessment of overall significance and can identify clusters of similar articles.

  QR Scanning Codes for the App

  Android

  iOS

4. ***Docphin***
   - ***Platforms***: iOS and Android
   - ***App Creator***: Docphin
   - ***Version***: 2.4.1
   - ***App Size***: 48.9 MB
   - ***App Icon***:

- ***App Screenshots***:

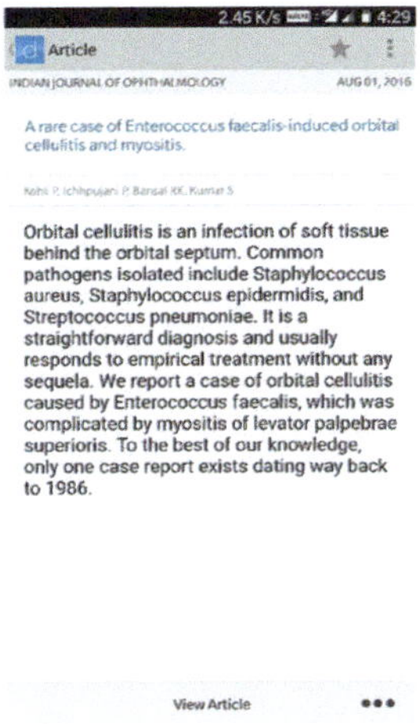

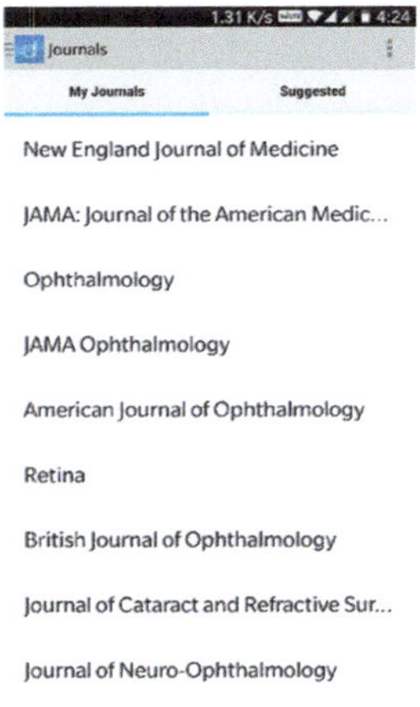

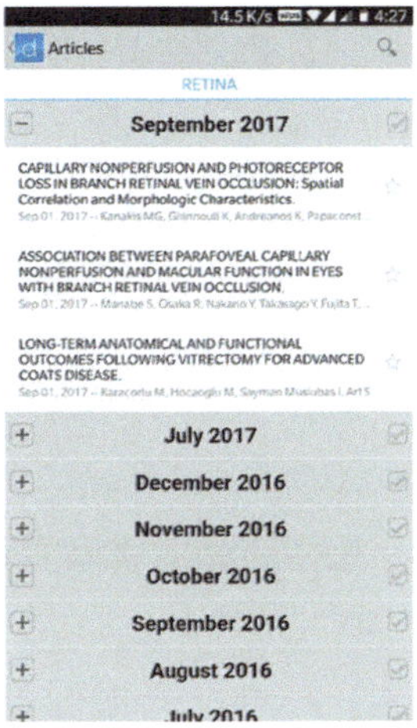

- ***Features***:
  This application provides an alternative way to read, organize and review PubMed articles. It makes it easy to follow one's chosen journals and access over 1000 landmark articles by speciality, topic or drug class. The app can help create an alert to track chosen topics or authors and also see which articles are trending in one's chosen speciality/subspeciality and among their peers. A personalized email is sent weekly which summarizes the trending articles in the chosen field and new content in the chosen journals. Additionally, the user can save articles to read later, organize them into folders and share the folders with colleagues. The app is free to use but requires a free Docphin account sign-up.

  QR Scanning Codes for the App

  Android iOS

5. ***PubMed Mobile and Pro*** *(Free, 2.99$)*
   - ***Platforms***: Android
   - ***App Creator***: CRinUS
   - ***Version***: 2.4.1
   - ***App Size***: 14 MB

- ***App Icon***:

- ***App Screenshots***:

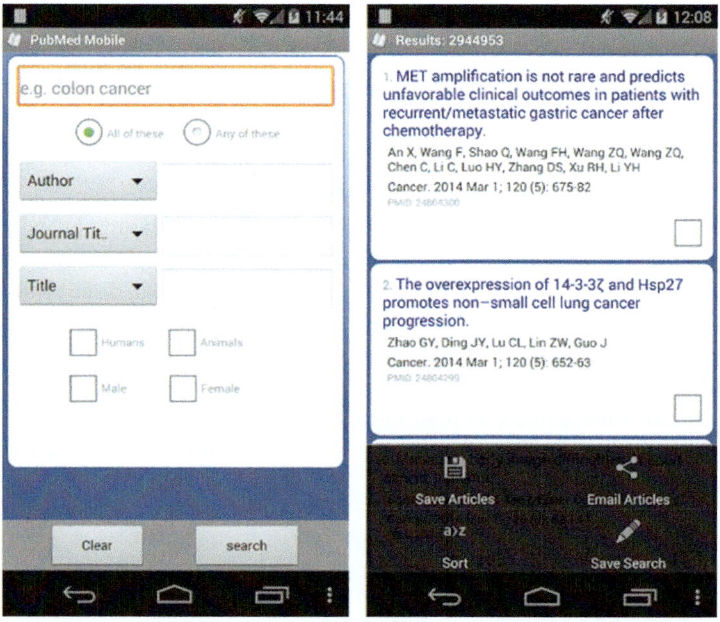

- ***Features***:
  This application offers a seamless experience to access PubMed content. The ability to search articles by author name requires an additional pro upgrade.

  QR Scanning Codes for the App

6. ***PubMed Hub*** *(Free and $1.99)*
   - ***Platforms***: Android and iOS
   - ***App Creator***: Omelette Inc
   - ***Version***: 1.1
   - ***App Size***: 1 MB
   - ***App Icon***:
   - ***App Screenshots***:

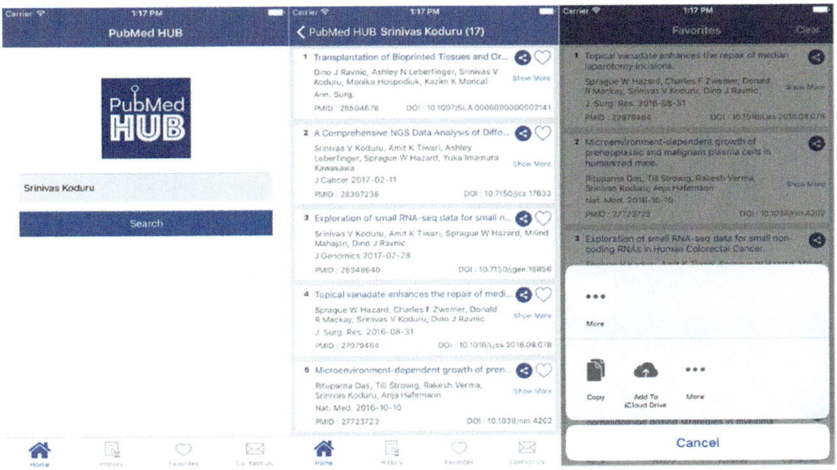

   - ***Features***:
     This application also helps to access PubMed content. The app has an interface that is easy to use, keyword searches display, chronological order, article title, author names, affiliations, journal name, year, volume, issue and page numbers along with PMID and DOI. Additionally, sharing is easily accessible, and one can select favourites for later reading.

- ***QR Scanning Codes for the App***

Android iOS

7. ***UptoDate***
   - ***Platforms***: iOS and Android
   - ***App Creator***: Wolters Kluwer
   - ***Version***: 2.30
   - ***App Size***: 22.9 MB
   - ***App Icon***:

   - ***App Screenshots***:

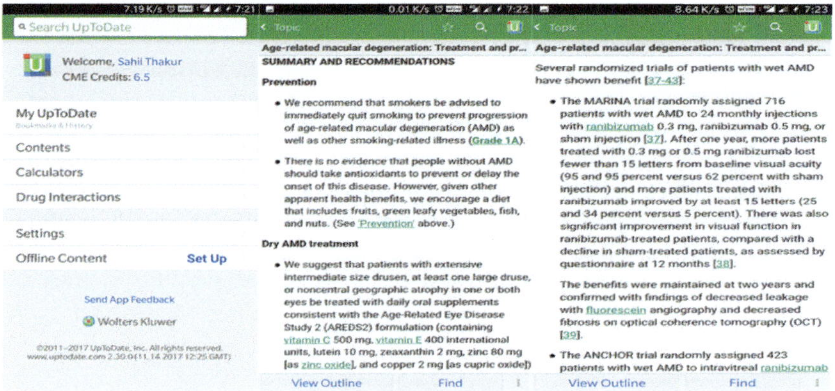

- ***Features***:
  UpToDate is an evidence-based reliable clinical resource with healthcare information including drug topics and recommendations. It is a subscription-based service, and institutional access is available in most of the medical institutes across the world. The application has been the focus of several research studies that evaluate increasing use of mobile technology in health-care. In a study by Wallace et al., 77% users indicated willingness to change a treatment plan based on the application recommendations [2]. There is how-ever dearth of content on ophthalmology currently on the UpToDate application but we see that being addressed in the near future by the application publisher.

  QR Scanning Codes for the App

  Android

  iOS

Additionally, there are resources available across software platforms that can help gather data from resources like Scopus, Google Scholar, Open Athens, Shibboleth and borderline legal platforms like LibGen. These are however less interactive, require subscription fee and are difficult to navigate using the current available tools. For research in resource-limited countries, a combination of the tools described above and institutional login access to Hinari are often more than enough to facilitate easy intuitive access to scientific research from around the world.

References

1. Barjak F. Research productivity in the internet era. Scientometrics. 2006;68(3):343–60.
2. Wallace KL, Beckett RD, Sheehan AH. Pharmacist perception and use of UpToDate®. J Med Libr Assoc. 2014;102(4):296–300.

Smartphones and Telemedicine in Ophthalmology

11

Telemedicine screening in ophthalmology usually involves the remote gathering of images, anterior segment and fundus photographs, with subsequent analysis to identify patients who have a referral-warranted ocular disease.

Screening can be done for several ophthalmic diseases, salient being diabetic retinopathy, age-related macular degeneration, retinopathy of prematurity and glaucoma.

A. **Diabetic Retinopathy**

The pandemic of diabetes is on the rise across the globe and so is its dreaded complication, diabetic retinopathy (DR). The gold standard for diagnosing DR is 7-field stereoscopic-dilated fundus photographs graded by the modified Airlie House classification protocol by trained photographers doing specialized film processing and archiving [1]. This is logistically not possible for screening the population. Hence, single-field digital fundus photography has been adopted as a modality to screen the masses. The number of patients with diabetes is growing exponentially; the only way to potentially screen all of these patients for DR would be to involve non-eye care professionals through access to telemedicine. Traditionally nonmydriatic and mydriatic fundus photography has been used for screening purpose, but the currently available smartphones, having cameras with resolution of 5 megapixels and better, are providing high-quality images, with and without adapters. The option of zooming on the smartphone touch-screen to enlarge the images for better visualization is an added advantage.

Tools: Some apps for mobile retinal imaging have been covered in the chapter on Apps and Social Networking Pages for Retinal Diseases. A few additional tools and apps are discussed here.

1. ***Magnifi Photoadapter for iPhone***

   Magnifi photoadapter connects the camera on an iPhone to an optical instrument with an eyepiece (binoculars, microscopes, telescopes, etc.) allowing the healthcare professional to take images and record videos through the eyepiece.

P. Ichhpujani, S. Thakur, *Smart Resources in Ophthalmology*, Current Practices in Ophthalmology, https://doi.org/10.1007/978-981-13-0140-7_11

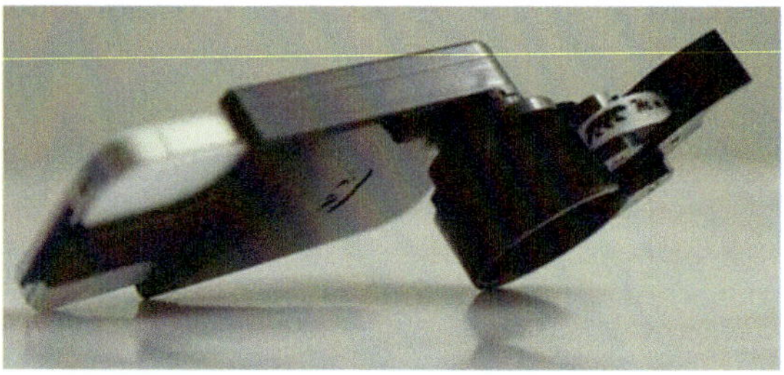

Site URL: http://www.arcturuslabs.com

2. **iExaminer PanOptic Ophthalmoscope**

   The iExaminer includes a panoptic portable ophthalmoscope that is more portable than a slit lamp but requires the purchase of a panoptic unit and the skill to use a direct ophthalmoscope. Additionally, easy and instantaneous sharing of images is not possible.

   Site URL: https://www.welchallyn.com/content/welchallyn/americas/en/microsites/iexaminer.html

   Welch Allyn iExaminer Pro App:

   - ***Platforms***: iOS (iPhone and iPad)
   - ***App Creator:*** *Welch Allyn, Inc.*
   - ***Version:*** *1.1*
   - ***App Size:*** *2.2 MB*
   - ***App Icon***:

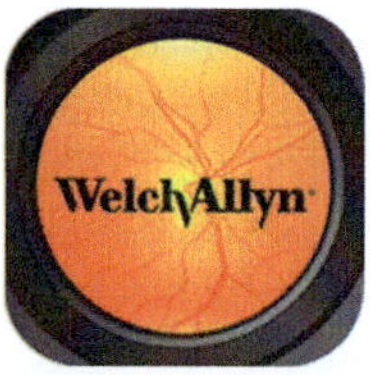

   - ***App Screenshot***:

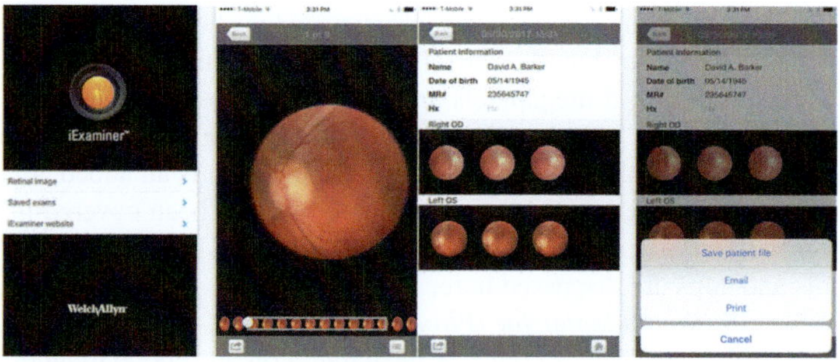

   - ***Features***:

     This app is used in conjunction with the Welch Allyn iExaminer adapter. Welch Allyn PanOptic Ophthalmoscope can be attached to select iPhone models to capture, store and retrieve fundus images. It also allows emailing and printing of patient files.

QR Scanning Code of the App

3. ***VOLK iNview***

   The Volk iNview is an innovative new ophthalmic camera device able to capture wide-angle (50°) digital colour images of the fundus using an Apple iPhone or iPod.

   Site URL: https://volk.com/index.php/volk-products/ophthalmic-cameras/volk-inview.html

   VOLK iNview:

   - ***Platforms***: iOS (iPhone and iPad)
   - ***App Creator***: Volk Optical, Inc.
   - ***Version***: 1.5.0
   - ***App Size***: 4.3 MB
   - ***App Icon***:

   - ***App Screenshots***:

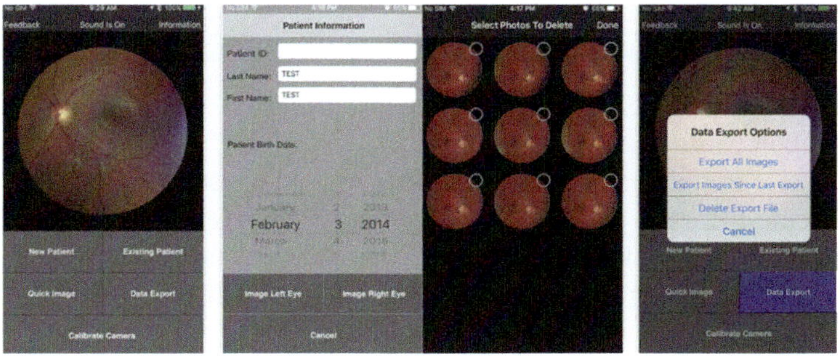

   - ***Features***

     This app used along with the Volk iNview retinal imaging attachment is easy to use for obtaining retinal images for purposes of general visualization, patient education and record retention. iNview uses patented auto-capture technology that eliminates the need for operators to

manually capture images. All patient data and images are encrypted within the application. Even if the iOS device is lost or stolen, the patient data within the application remains secure without the passkey.
QR Scanning Code for the App

4. ***EyePhotoDoc Adapter***
Although this adapter allows for high-quality imaging, it requires a slit lamp, not allowing its use outside of ophthalmology clinics as a screening tool. But if a peripheral health centre has a slit lamp, then this adapter allows capturing high-resolution images (8–12 Megapixel) and HD/UHD videos. The photos are then integrated into the patient's Electronic Health Records.

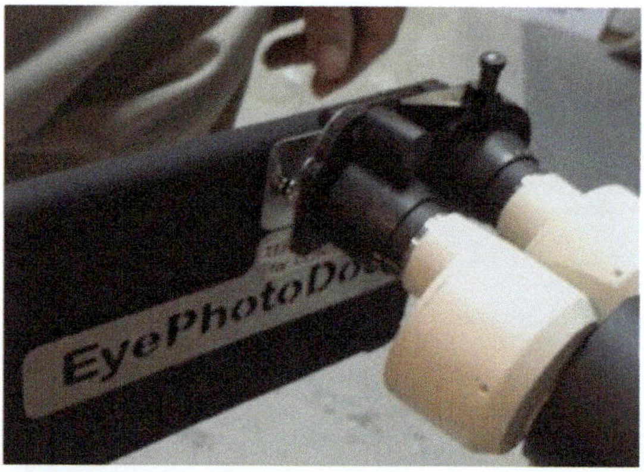

Site URL: http://www.eyephotodoc.com

5. ***Paxos Suite***
Paxos product suite by DigiSight is a cloud-based portal that creates an outcome-focussed patient profile from data procured from multiple sources. It involves use of Checkup study, an app that checks multiple vision parameters and has a dynamic Amsler grid and Paxos Mobile, a mobile application that allows the screening team to capture ophthalmic photographs of patients anywhere [2].
Checkup study:
   - ***Platforms***: iOS (iPhone and iPad)
   - ***App Creator***: Digisight Technologies

- ***Version***: 1.7.12
- ***App Size***: 10.7 MB
- ***App Icon***:

- ***App Screenshot***:

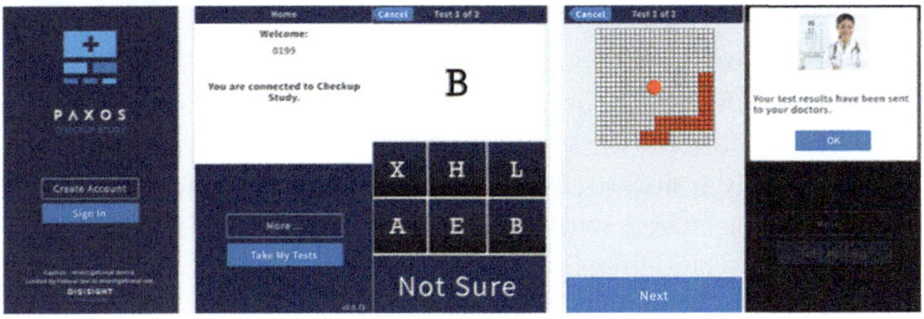

- ***Features***:
  The app enables patients to test their visual function at home on a smart device (supported iPod, iPhone, or iPad) and share their test results automatically and securely with their physicians.

  QR Scanning Code for the App

Paxos Mobile:

- ***Platforms***: iOS (iPhone and iPad)
- ***App Creator***: DigiSight Technologies
- ***Version***: 1.7.12
- ***App Size***: 10.7 MB
- ***App Icon***:

- ***App Screenshots***:

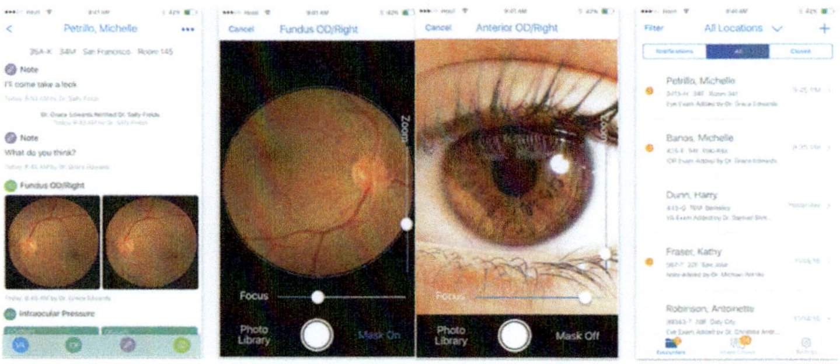

- ***Features***:
Paxos Mobile enables healthcare professionals to capture high-resolution photos of the eye at the point of care. Captured photos are instantaneously transmitted and stored in the Paxos cloud and can be analysed later or shared with experts. This software meets HIPPA security and privacy guidelines.

QR Scanning Code for the App

The Paxos Mobile application can be used in conjunction with the Paxos Scope smartphone adapter (previously known as EyeGo), which converts a mobile device into an ophthalmic camera. This clinical photographs taken with this attachment have shown a high level of agreement with those taken with existing clinic cameras (92.6% anterior, 84.4% posterior) [3].

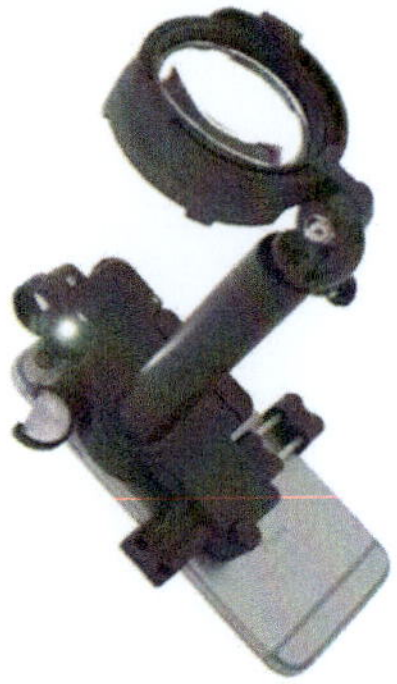

6. ***D-EYE 2.0***
    - ***Platforms***: iOS (iPhone and iPad)
    - ***App Creator***: D-EYE SRL
    - ***Version***: 2.1.16
    - ***App Size***: 38.7 MB
    - ***App Icon***:
    - ***App Screenshots***:

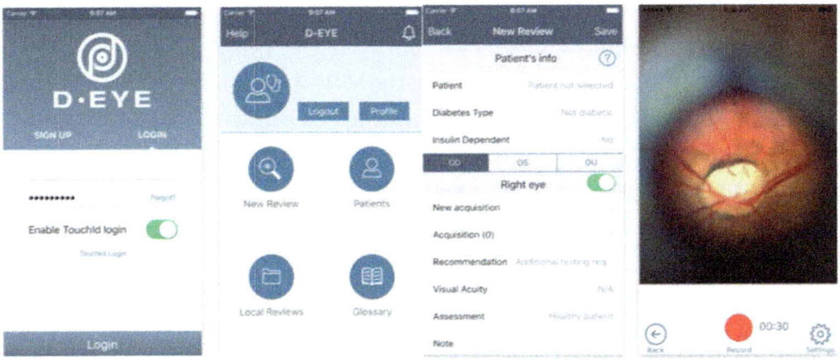

    - ***Features***:
    The D-EYE lens with the app is an eye health screening tool using a smartphone. Ophthalmologists, optometrists, neurologists and even paediatricians are using it to record a retinal exam capturing 'direct' images or video of the posterior pole (without the condensing lens) that can be shared with colleagues for further assessment and saved to a patient file for future reference. D-EYE uses light from the smartphone, which is off axis from the phone's camera aperture, to illuminate the interior of the eye for examination while eliminating corneal glare.
    In a comparative study of 120 patients, D-EYE was reported to be highly sensitive in detection of DR when a retina specialist viewed the fundus at the point of care through a dilated pupil [4].

    QR Scanning Code for the App

B. **Age-Related Macular Degeneration (AMD)**
Given the aging global population, the prevalence of AMD is increasing. Retina image screening using smartphones is therefore seen as beneficial in identification of people with early-stage AMD. Early detection will help in designing preventative strategies for late AMD.

PEEK Retina and D-EYE can prove to be good tele-health solutions for detecting AMD.

C. **Retinopathy of Prematurity (ROP)**
Retinopathy of prematurity is a major cause of childhood blindness.

Studies have shown that ROP also affects infants cared for in smaller, rural locations, exploding the age-old myth that it is restricted to tertiary care urban centres [5, 6]. With this background, Karnataka Internet Assisted Diagnosis of Retinopathy of Prematurity (KIDROP), India's first and now the world's largest telemedicine network to tackle infant blindness from ROP, came into being [7].

The infant screening is done by taking retinal images using portable wide-field retinal digital camera (Retcam). These images are graded by experts and management decisions while in the NICU (i.e. discharge; screen again and when; urgent referral to an ophthalmologist required) are conveyed to the attending doctor. Images captured by the graders are also uploaded and read on the smartphones of ROP specialists in the city or elsewhere on a customized platform.

D. **Glaucoma**
Glaucoma remains largely asymptomatic in the early stage and is noticed by the patient once irreversible field loss has occurred. It has been seen that >50% of individuals are unaware of diagnosis until glaucoma reaches an advanced stage.

In developing countries like India, people residing in rural or remote areas have limited access to trained ophthalmologists who can detect early glaucomatous signs. Therefore, smartphone-based teleophthalmology for glaucoma screening is critical for early diagnosis and treatment.

Smartphone ophthalmoscopy has shown substantial agreement with slit lamp examination for the estimation of vertical cup to disc ratio [8].

Non-clinical photographers have used the Peek Retina adapter and smartphone to acquire optic nerve images at a standard that enabled comparable independent remote grading of the images to those acquired using a desktop retinal camera operated by an ophthalmic assistant [9].

With the available evidence, it seems smartphones will undoubtedly be on the forefront of screening retinal diseases in coming years. Technological improvements that enable peripheral visualization of the fundus, standardization of image capture and improved camera hardware and software will facilitate improvement in smartphone fundus photography.

References

1. Rajalakshmi R, Arulmalar S, Usha M, et al. Validation of smartphone-based retinal photography for diabetic retinopathy screening. PLoS One. 2015;10:e0138285.
2. Toy BC, Myung DJ, He L, et al. Smartphone-based dilated fundus photography and near visual acuity testing as inexpensive screening tools to detect referral warranted diabetic eye disease. Retina. 2016;36(5):1000–8.
3. Ludwig CA, Murthy SI, Pappuru RR, et al. A novel smartphone ophthalmic imaging adapter: user feasibility studies in Hyderabad, India. Indian J Ophthalmol. 2016;64(3):191–200.
4. Russo A, Morescalchi F, Costagliola C, Delcassi L, Semeraro F. Comparison of smartphone ophthalmoscopy with slit-lamp biomicroscopy for grading diabetic retinopathy. Am J Ophthalmol. 2015;159(2):360–4.
5. Hungi B, Vinekar A, Datti N, et al. Retinopathy of prematurity in a rural neonatal intensive care unit in South India—a prospective study. Indian J Pediatr. 2012;79:911–5.
6. Vinekar A. IT-enabled innovation to prevent infant blindness in rural India: the KIDROP experience. J Indian Bus Res. 2011;3:98–102.
7. Vinekar A, Gilbert C, Dogra M, et al. The KIDROP model of combining strategies for providing retinopathy of prematurity screening in underserved areas in India using wide-field imaging, tele-medicine, non-physician graders and smart phone reporting. Indian J Ophthalmol. 2014;62(1):41–9.
8. Russo A, Mapham W, Turano R, et al. Comparison of smartphone ophthalmoscopy with slit-lamp biomicroscopy for grading vertical cup-to-disc ratio. J Glaucoma. 2016;25(9):e777–81.
9. Bastawrous A, Giardini ME, Bolster NM, et al. Clinical validation of smartphone based adapter: peek retina for optic disc imaging in Kenya. JAMA Ophthalmol. 2016;134(2):151–8.

Index

P. Ichhpujani, S. Thakur, *Smart Resources in Ophthalmology*, Current Practices in Ophthalmology, https://doi.org/10.1007/978-981-13-0140-7

CPI Antony Rowe
Eastbourne, UK
August 06, 2019